N.E. McMORRAN

MOOJAG

and the SLOTH GUARDIANS

SPONDYLUXPRESS

First published December 2025 in the UK by Spondylux Press.
Spondylux Press empowers creatives to thrive on their own terms and enables publishers to produce inclusive, affirmative content through neurodivergent consulting, mentoring, and editing services.
www.spondyluxpress.com

Editors: Catalina Gutierrez, Jax Blunt.

Cover art by Abi Stevens 2025
Illustration on Page 10 by Chiaki Kamikawa 2020

ISBN: 978-1-8380978-4-4 (Print)
ISBN: 978-1-8380978-5-1 (E-book)
ISBN: 978-1-8380978-2-0 (Audiobook - 'Moojag and the Auticode Secret')

A CIP catalogue record for this title is available from the British Library.
Printed and bound by Clays Ltd in the UK, using sustainably sourced, manufactured, and FSC certified paper.

Praise for MOOJAG and the SLOTH GUARDIANS

DANIEL AUBREY
Author *Dark Island*

'A brilliant, important, and exhilarating final instalment in the award-winning cli-fi series. As someone who has ADHD, I know all too well what it's like to be called lazy when you're anything but, and when you're just trying to protect yourself from overwhelm, and the analogy of the sloths works perfectly. I wish I'd had this book as a kid, and if I had young children, this series would be top of the pile of books I'd be reading to them. A vital read for anyone, not just ND folk or people with neurodivergent kids. Such a fitting finale to a wonderful series—I cannot recommend it highly enough.'

JAX BLUNT *@liveotherwise*
Neurodivergent Advocate, Writer, Home Educator

'I loved returning to Moojag's world of science and mystery. Familiar characters band together to stave off a new villanous plot and rescue endangered animals, all while spreading a message of empathy and inclusion across generations and neurotypes. A great yarn with an important message.'

CATALINA GUTIERREZ
Editor, Writer

'I adore the sloth motif, for the cute factor and the likeness to how neurodivergent people go at their own pace: it shows the struggles that come with operating differently to others. There is whimsy abound and appreciation of the power of bringing understanding to a world that isn't easy to navigate. The strings of PIE's history are pulled together, and the ending feels very natural. When I read a Moojag book, I always wish I could have a Gajoomstik plushie, and then remember they just look like sticks of rock.'

Praise for MOOJAG and the SLOTH GUARDIANS

WILLIAM VANDERPUYE
Director **Autistic Inclusive Meets**, Autistic Advocate

'An imaginative, magnificent, and deeply insightful futuristic adventure that crowns the series. I am full of admiration and praise for its positive representation and abundance of fantastic ideas. The book draws a powerful, masterful allegory using the endangered sloth. This insight creates a powerful parallel for neurodivergent individuals like myself. Expertly using the interplay between humour and suspense, the narrative encapsulates the value of difference... This thrilling story, that captivates the reader's interest and attention at the turn of each page, spreads a profound message of empathy and inclusion across all neurotypes, affirming that different is good and delivering both 'fantastical fun' and peril. Though the story is primarily aimed at children, I strongly feel that its message is very relevant to our world given our current socio-economic and political climate. I'd give it a 10/10!'

DR CHRIS PAPADOPOULOS
Author *Voices of Neurodiversity: An Inclusive Encyclopaedia*
Founder **London Autism Group Charity**

'Right from the opening pages, I was captivated. McMorran's writing is highly immersive and vivid... The worldbuilding is genuinely original and inventive... clever sci-fi. The voice of the narrator is warm, funny, authentic and easy to read. But I think what resonates most is the sloth metaphor at the heart of the story... A lot of neurodivergent people will feel very seen and validated through this. I also value the push to celebrate a world where we are free to be our true, authentic selves. There isn't anything more important than that and this book promotes this message in a clever, fun, original way that isn't heavy handed. Overall, an imaginative, affirming story with heart and originality.'

Read the full reviews, and more, at **MOOJAG.COM**

Letter from the author

Welcome to *Sloth Guardians,* the last adventure in the MOOJAG series! I made sloths the heroes in this story because the cute but endangered creatures have a surprising amount in common with us humans, especially neurodivergent folk. You see, sloths are very much misunderstood, with a false reputation for being lazy. But the real reason they're so slow is that they're saving all their energy for important tasks like processing food, staying safe, and protecting the rainforest! They're highly sensitive, too, so they need their space. They wear a mask that makes it seem like they're smiling, even when they're afraid or in pain, and they freeze when they're threatened. Writing this book, I realised that none of us are lazy; we're simply surviving in a world that doesn't always understand or make time for us.

I hope you enjoy it. Don't forget to follow us and tell all your friends about Moojag!

@MOOJAGbook @nemcmorran

info@moojag.com
www.moojag.com

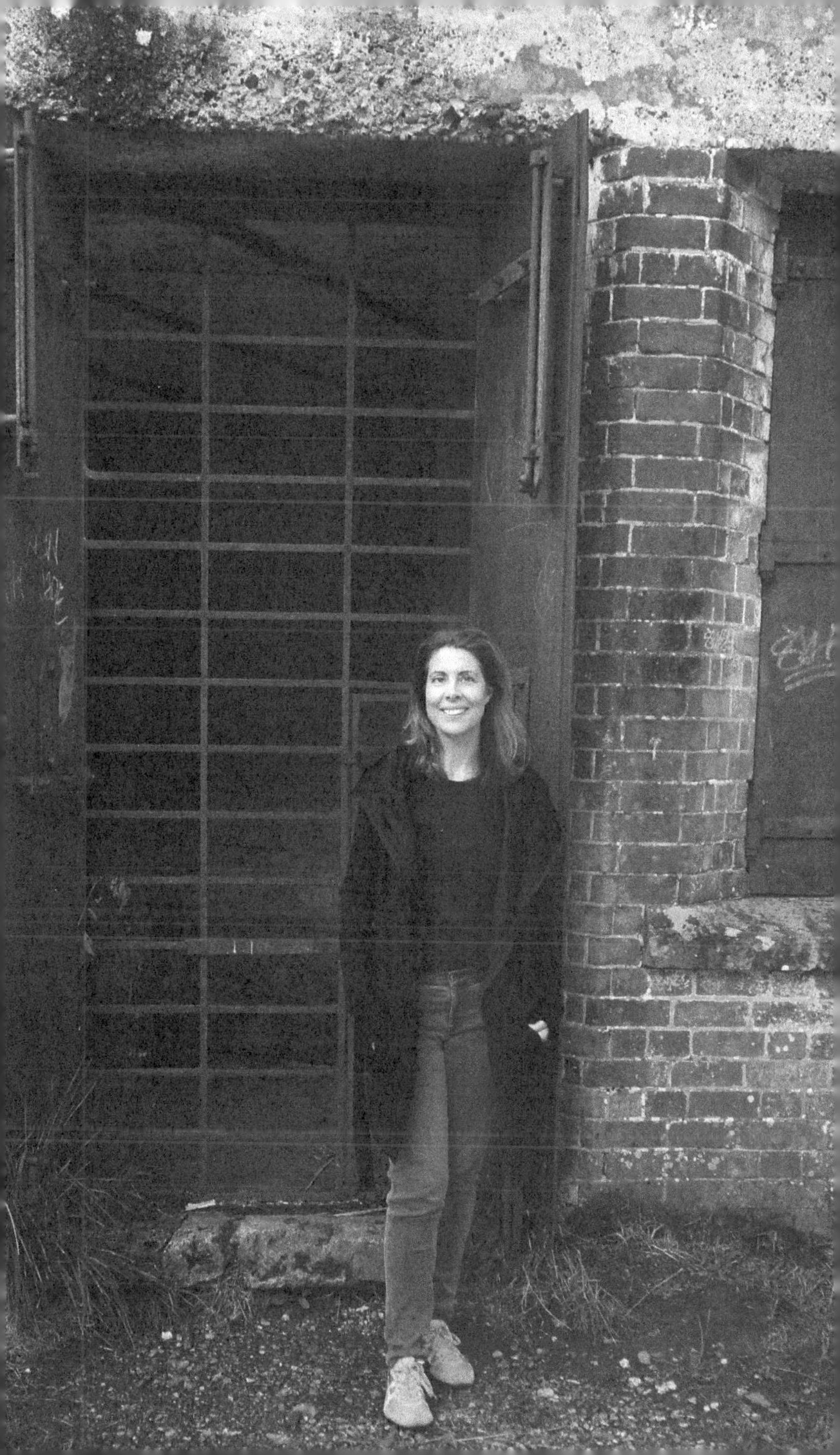

Dedicated to my gumptious grans:
Margaret (d. 1995), Tessi (d. 2023), and *ma belle* Marcelle.

And in loving memory of Ben

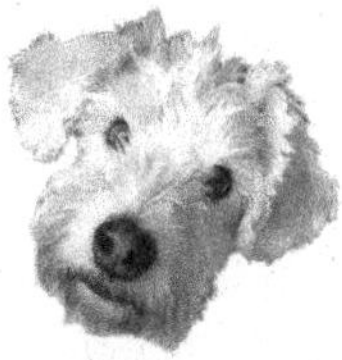

Thanks to editors, Catalina Gutierrez and Jax Blunt; artist, Abi Stevens; Chris, James, and friends at LAG, and all who have reviewed and supported the 'Sloth Guardians'.

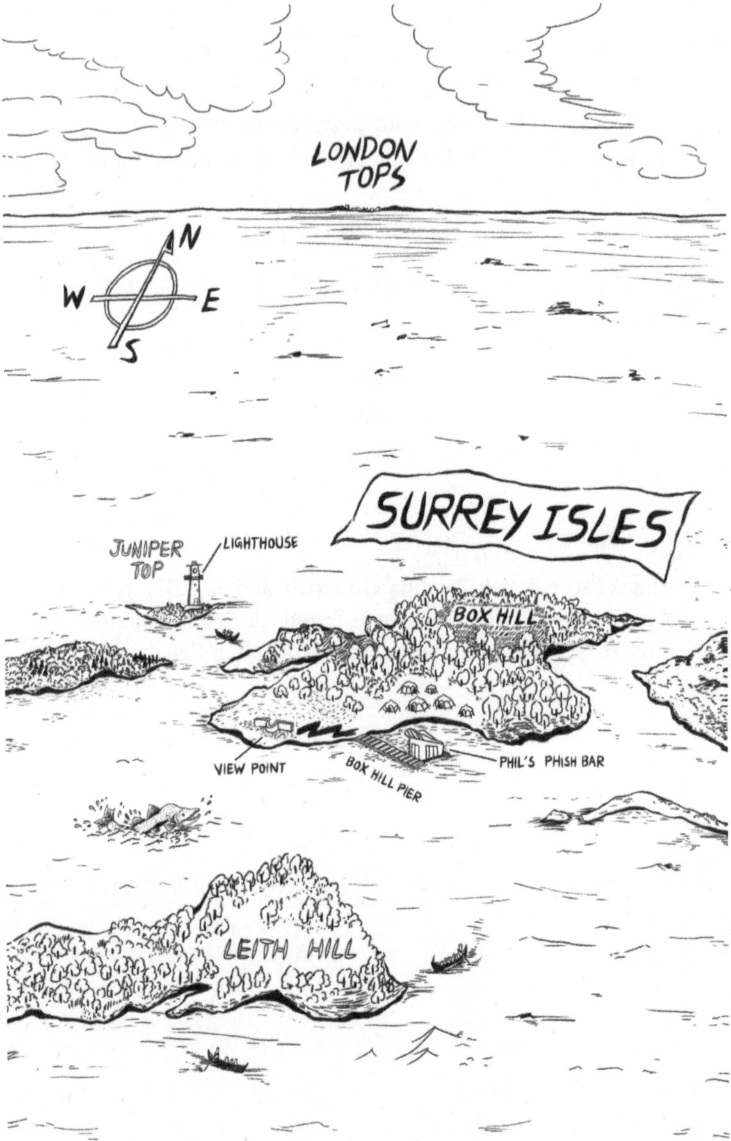
LONDON TOPS
N
W
E
S
SURREY ISLES
JUNIPER TOP
LIGHTHOUSE
BOX HILL
VIEW POINT
BOX HILL PIER
PHIL'S PHISH BAR
LEITH HILL

This is the sequel to 'Moojag and the Lost Memories'…

Ten years ago, in 2044, when I was only three, a gigantic tidal wave swept Britain. The 'Great Surge' sunk even more of England, after years of flooding, and turned its highest points into lots of smaller islands. London became London Tops and the Surrey Hills became Surrey Isles. When it got too difficult living on Hampstead Top, without enough land to grow real food, we moved to Box Hill Island in the Surrey Isles. We'd lost Mum and my brother Monzi already, so it was just me, Dad, and Gran. They created the 'Real World': a community of neurodivergents—people who think and feel things differently—living outdoors with the help of our PIEs and 3D printers.

"What are PIEs?" I hear you ask? No, pre-Surgers, they're not stuffed pastries! Before Gran founded the Real World, she invented our amazing solar-charged, full-body electronic skin, complete with a single Spondylux shell device. PIE is the computer we wear instead of clothes to protect us from all weathers and keep us safe from harm and disease. It does everything all your devices can do, too, like *whatsnapchatinstatwitface*. And it has some other incredible functions as well, that I still have no clue about!

We've been living the perfect life, free to be our true selves, ever since. Well, until Adam, Izzy, and I met Moojag, that is! Everything changed again when the outsider led us to Gajoomdom—a curious, sticky, underground world full of artificial sweets, inhabited by the Conqip group (a gang of nasty, smelly, greedy, controlling men); the Pofs (a race of small but super strong winged kids); the Auts (twenty-one autistic teen coders with super senses); and a bunch of Gajoomstiks (innocent candy-producing robots).

We found out that the Conqips were holding those kids captive, and plotting to destroy our home. Turned out, we were the only ones who could rescue everyone and save our Real World, too.

But when we figured out who Moojag really was, and he didn't come home with us, I had to go back down there to get him, only to discover three imprisoned super grans with memory loss. And one other very special person we thought was lost forever. Little did we know that the whole island was about to blow and our home was still in danger!

And that's how we ended up here, friends. So, keep reading to find out what on earth a bunch of sloths are doing on Box Hill and how, this time, saving the Real World is literally going to take guts!

If you haven't read the 'Auticode Secret' yet, check out the award-winning audiobook, too, read by a fabulous cast of neurodivergent actors, including narrators Indica Watson and Ria Lina.

1

L - A - Z - Y

A foghorn booms over the crashing waves as a flock of squawking seagulls sweeps out through the mist.

"Ahoy there!" bellows Captain Phil.

I raise my head from Mum's cosy tum to find her tired but happy face gazing back at me. Gran, our inflated-human-lifeboat gently rocking us over the swishing waves, points to the rescue ship. Now afloat beside us, it's smothered in ash and dotted with a thousand black dents from the Conqips' deadly explosion. Moojag's already up there on the bow with Dad. Captain Phil salutes us before throwing down a bundle of braided yellow rope. I lunge forward to catch the twisted snake as it swings straight for us and pass it to Gran. She drops its looped end over a hook attached to the back of her puffed-up hood. "Grab tight, you two!" she shouts, before giving Phil and Moojag the thumbs up. They haul us up out of the water and onto the slippery wooden slats of Old Myrta.

Moojag and Phil bow to each other, while I jump up to give Dad one big long hug. I catch him glance at Moojag, eyes glazed over. He looks sad and happy all at once. It must be strange for them, seeing each other again after all these years. Mum, too. Gran pulls back her hood, deflating the PIE skin and blasting a whoosh of air through Mum's dull salt-and-pepper hair.

Gran places an arm around Mum's shoulder and turns to Dad with a wink. "Look who we found down there," she says, waving to the small mountain of blown-up-island rubble in the distance. The lighthouse beacon is all that remains of Juniper Island, plopped on top like a pre-Surge cake decoration. Dad nods to Mum and she nods back, but then both quickly look away. I stare out in either direction, but there's nothing there. Gran grips my hand; Moojag's too. "We made it!" she declares, lifting up our arms. "Safe and sound."

Safe, maybe, but too much sound for my liking. Moojag rescues his hand and presses a finger to his lips. I nod back as Gran finally lets go of mine.

"Nice cup of tea, anyone?" asks Dad.

This is no time for tea, Dad. What about the

Conqips? "What about Box Hill?" I ask, hunching my shoulders. What makes a 'nice cup of tea', anyway?

Dad pouts at my bunched-up forehead. "What about those two crafty caterpillars on your face?" I squint back at him and cross my arms. He leans forward to brush my angry brows back into smooth arches with his thumb. The pressure against my supraorbitals feels good. *Supraorbital, supraorbital, supraorbital.* I swipe my hand over my forehead, removing all trace of Dad's finger, and take a step back. Moojag nudges me and points to a curled-up figure on the far deck—an old man in a suit sat with his head between his knees. Miserable Uncle Aldon.

"*Supraorbital.*" Oh, did I say that out loud?

"*Non,*" says Moojag, shaking his head. "*Oncle* Aldon."

"Maybe you two can cheer him up," suggests Dad.

"You think?" I answer, brow raised.

"He's not a saint, I know," says Dad, placing his hand on my shoulder, "but it really seems like he's changed—for the better."

I pout back. "Maybe."

"Maybe *non,*" says Moojag, turning with a huff to check on Mum. She's resting on a chair beside Phil, looking even paler than when we found her in that cold, dark room down in Gajoomdom.

"You're right," says Dad. "Best get straight home."

If the Conqips get their way, there'll be no more Box Hill. Then where will 'home' be, Dad?

"Where the heart is," declares Moojag, with a twirl. He stabs his chest with a closed fist then pokes mine.

"Someone once sang," adds Dad, flicking Moojag's top hat as I shake my head, "wherever you lay your hat—that's your home…" Dad and his songs. It makes sense when our mysterious Beatles-loving friend Wats does it. Dad's just embarrassing.

"And if you don't have a hat?" I ask.

"I suppose," says Gran, stepping in as Moojag polishes his hat with his sleeve, "it means you should be content wherever you are, and make that your home."

I wonder if the Pofs have already made Box Hill *their* home. "How're they doing," I ask, as Phil steers the ship round for the pier, "the Auts and the Pofs?" I can just make out the boardwalk now. Someone's out there waving to us.

Dad frowns, squinting to see who it is. "Afraid we lost one," he says, glancing back at me.

"Oh no!" I say, copying his frown.

"Kitty up to mischief again," croaks Aldon. "Just like that tricky old mother of hers."

"When they arrived at Box Hill," explains Dad, "they were so distracted by all the colourful flowers and 'sweet fruits', they all went zooming off into the woods. We found them hanging off the Autumnalis tree, like a bunch of cheeky sloths. All but Kitty." Poor Pof.

"So they did," nods Phil. "But you're not to worry," he says, stroking his sparkly beard. "Either Kitty is well, or she is sick. But!" he adds, cocking his head and shaking a finger, "if she is indeed sick, there are only two things to worry about: either she will live, or truly she will die." Moojag's eyes widen. He tips his top hat and holds it flat against his chest. I hope she is not dead. "We'll find the little Might, though," he says finally, "to be sure."

I nod.

"Better not turn her back the right way up, when you do," exclaims Moojag, flipping his hat and somersaulting over me. "She may explode."

"Why would she explode?" I ask.

"That's what the Conqips used to say about the sloths in Gajoomdom."

"What were the Conqips doing with sloths!"

"Pets," he says, hands on hips and elbows sticking right out. I shake my head. "They only poop once a week."

"True," Gran confirms, nodding. "They get so constipated, they end up pooping a third of their body weight when they do go. Their swelling four-chambered bellies are full of gas, but they could never explode. Neither are they L-A-Z-Y." 'Lazy' must be another word she left out of the Brave New Dictionary.

"That's why they're called sloths," says Moojag.

"Yes," she says, raising her voice, "but because they're *not* L-A-Z-Y, not because they are!" She squints, looking out to sea. "When are we going back home, to London Tops? ...How old did you say I was?"

"As young as you feel, Nem Avti," answers Mum. "Isn't that what you used to say?"

Gran nods back at her with a smile.

"You see," explains Dad, combing through Gran's silky silver hair with his fingers, "hundreds of years ago, when people first spotted the grinning, monkey-like creatures hanging out in the trees all the time, they assumed the furry things slept all day. But sloths don't sleep much at all—they're just busy saving all their energy."

"Super smart, sensitive beings," adds Mum.

People didn't get them, then? Just like us neurodivergents, before the Great Surge.

Gran nods at my frowning face. "Slow doesn't mean weak or L-A-Z-Y—it's a survival strategy!"

"Never stress out a sloth," warns Dad, shaking his head. "They're likely to lash out and attack."

"Five minutes to dock," calls Phil, with the ship closing in on the port and the figure we saw before coming into focus: a bald-headed man in a suit.

"Not an RW," Dad whispers to Gran.

"A Conqip, dear," she shouts, firmly patting his shoulder, as Moojag leaps behind me.

"*Ugh*," mutters Aldon. "Crusty Lord Moneybags' beaten us to it, has he?" Mum's slender hand reaches out for mine and grips it tight, while Gran grabs my other hand and squeezes it even harder!

We watch, open-mouthed, as Brix strides up to the mooring with a small girl cradled in the crook of his arm. A Pof wearing a sparkling orange PIE skin that has perfectly moulded around all her beautiful curves. "*Au revoir* to the stupid Real World," he hollers up, "you lazy little nerds!"

2

CONQIP INVASION

Where are all the Real Worlders? What has he done with all our friends?!

"Well, don't just stand there," shouts Brix, ordering us off the ship. "Get down here *right* now and hand over your crazy PIE suits to Orange Pof. Do exactly as she says and don't even *think* about disappearing."

Dad steps out first onto the boardwalk and looks Brix straight in the eye. "What have you done now, little Con?"

Brix curls his lip and sniggers. "I'm not *done* yet!"

"Have you seen my girlfriends?" asks Gran, turning to the fidgety Pof hovering beside her. "Stella? Sophia?"

Brix just grunts and stomps off. Orange Pof glares at Gran, then leans in to sniff her. "You smell, WB1," she says, wrinkling up her nose. She must've gotten so used to the scent of urine that she smells it even when it's not there. "You're walking!" she adds, digging her fists into her hips.

"Of course I am," says Gran, gazing into the Pof's beady little eyes as though she's lost something in them. "I sing and dance too! Would you like me to—"

Orange Pof grabs Gran's arm and whisks her off the ship. "Come on, Real Nerders," she calls back to us. "Must deliver you to your lodgings, now. You too, Aut-Pof," she adds, bowing to Moojag hovering beside her.

Dad takes Gran's hand, but she snatches it back and gives him a mean stare. "I can do it, man." She turns to me and whispers, "Who's that guy?"

"It's all right. It's only Dad. I mean, your son, Jack." She swivels back to scan his face and wobbles, swinging round to inspect mine, too, before warily offering back her hand. I hook Mum's arm inside mine and we step cautiously down off Myrta, followed at last by a tutting, hobbling Uncle Aldon. "Where are all the Real Worlders?" I ask the Pof spinning big, bright orange halos over our heads as she zooms round us in circles.

She grins, pausing for a moment in front of my face. "The real-fruit lizards?"

"Yes, the PIE-wearing people who live here?"

"*We* live here now. Your funny friends are waiting in *there*," she says, pointing to Phil's Phish Bar. She dishes out t-shirts with Brix's head printed on them for us to wear and snatches our PIE skins from us. "We're confiscating *all* skins," she exclaims, whizzing off, "until my *gorgeous* Darling Brix decides what to do with you all. Can't have you vanish into thin air again, can we!"

Phil dashes on ahead to his cherished bar, now packed with neurodivergent prisoners. He tugs at the heavy wooden door, but it's triple-locked.

Orange Pof chuckles, crossing her arms and sticking her nose up in the air. "You can't get in, beard man."

"We're in here!" shouts a boy.

"Adam?" I call at the frosted glass window. "Who's in there?"

"We're *all* in here."

"*Everyone*?"

"All the Real Worlders! And all the Super Auts too." No Pofs in there, then. So the Conqips are still using the little Mights to pull off their evil plans. Does he have Kitty, too, or is she actually lost?

"Freezin' in 'ere," cries a girl. "They got our PIEs, and we've eaten all the Frankenfish already!" Phil raises a bushy brow and turns to me with a wink. Izzy!

"Nem!" calls Adam. "We can barely move!"

"I demand to see the manager!" shrieks an older voice.

"Eggs 'n' cheese for me, please," yelps another.

"It won't take the weight much longer," says Phil, inspecting the bar's sagging deck.

"Over there!" says Orange Pof, pointing to the small floating hut moored alongside the bar. "No time for any of your nerd nonsense—I'm due my chocolate orange!" She pokes Phil's shoulder and ushers us all to the hut, before shoving everyone inside and clamping the doors closed behind us. Then the sound of a lock—no, two locks—no, three—clicking shut!

"How did he get them all in there?" asks Phil, peeking at his bar through a gap in the boards.

"He got us in here pretty easily," I say, arms crossed.

"What could we do?" he adds. "No point picking fights with a Conqip, or those muscly Pofs. Looks like they could do a lot of damage."

I nod.

"And anyway," continues Phil, "there's only seven of us, and hundreds of them next door."

"Only one way," answers Moojag, bouncing into us. "Sticky Gajooms."

I smile and clasp my hands. "Yes! They must have saved those brilliant robots, after all."

Gran sighs and shakes her head. "Poor sticks of rock, always being roped into evil Conqip plans."

"And Wats and Biermont?" I ask.

Dad nods. "Still on the Isle of Brix."

Aldon shakes his head and lets out a grunt. It tastes of disappointment, maybe a pinch of fear too. "They stayed behind with the Peace Gajooms to deal with the Conqips' dynamite," he groans.

"At least they're safe," I say with a shrug, laying Mum down on one of the inflated mats in the corner and covering her with another. She doesn't seem bothered. After being locked up for so long in Gajoomdom, this all probably just feels normal.

"Well," says Dad, peeking out through the wooden slats with Gran, "here's hoping they're safe!"

I hope so, too.

"Me three," adds Moojag with a twirl.

3

DOG NUT

I cover my ears at the doors clapping each time the wind whirls past the hut and hisses through the gap in the slats. I wish I had PIE to turn off all the noise. The hullabaloo. The racket. The ruckus. No. Stop!

Across the room, on a shelf—a black metal box. Hmm, what was it Gran kept in that thing..? I pull it down and let it slump to the floor.

"NERDERS!" Who the twit-face is that, now? "This is Conqip II speaking."

"Travis," utters Aldon, "what the devil are you two playing at?"

"We're going to get what we deserve, A'! And you, old man, aren't getting any of it." Aldon smirks at Gran and shakes his head. Like a clone, she does the same right back at him.

"A whack in the head?" Aldon answers, grabbing hold of a bent slat to pull himself up. "That's the least you deserve, you pathetic little phoney."

Everything goes quiet and Dad's eyes shoot sideways for the door, as though he's expecting Travis to bolt right in. But he doesn't. Gran isn't bothered, sat between us as she fiddles with the coded padlock on the box. Phil stands with his rugged body pressed against the wall, arms crossed behind his back. Mum is now fast asleep—too used to the sound of brawling Conqips.

"Once we get what we want," says Travis, "your Nerdivergents will work for us, or else they can jolly well diverge some place else. I hear Cyprus used to be very nice. Quiet. Very *slow*," he adds with a cackle. "They'd like it there. Sunny, too. Good for those stupid solar panels you love so."

Gran's head bolts up. "Please, someone make that man stop."

"What's the old bat saying?" splutters Travis. "She's M-A-D, I tell you. Well, I've more important things to do than talk to lessers such as she. Laters, alligators."

No. We need that door open! "Travis!" I call.

"That's my name—don't wear it out!"

"I heard you like doughnuts?"

The Conqip's lips smack so loud at the thought, we all hear it. "I wouldn't say no…"

"Moojag has one," I say, nodding to my brother shaking his head at me. "Just pretend," I whisper.

"*Oui*," he says, winking at me, "I indeed have a dog-nut." Dog-nut? Maybe it's so hard saying something untrue, that he has to create his own new words. They sound similar, at least.

CLINK, goes the first lock.

CLUNK, goes the second.

CLANK, goes the third, with Travis creeping in.

He pushes his middle against the door, slamming it shut, and as he stretches his arm to hold out the palm of his hand his hairy navel peeks through the gap in his shirt.

"Idiot," Aldon utters. Gran tuts at him while Travis throws back his head and pulls a comb from his jacket pocket to reshape his flopped quiff.

I step up to him and wave Dad over, too. "Did you know," I say, "in America, they ate over ten billion doughnuts a year?"

Dad nods, gesturing to Moojag. "They practically

lived off the old oil cakes."

"I bet you didn't know," says Gran, shaking her head at Travis, "doughnuts were first brought to the US by the Dutch. But the 'oly-koeks' were originally a treat for people who couldn't afford sugar and flour."

"Was a ship captain, invented the holes in 'em," adds Phil, stroking his beard.

"Prefer the jam-filled ones, myself," says Travis, wide-eyed.

"Like this one?" asks Moojag, throwing an invisible dog-nut to Gran pretending to catch it.

"It's yours..." she calls, cradling the invisible cake, as the panting, drooling man wanders over, "*if* you can spell 'doughnut'."

While Travis busily searches for the dog-nut and desperately attempts to spell, Moojag pulls me up onto his shoulders. Dad gently releases the door for us and we hover out.

"I'll give you a clue, shall I?" says Gran's fading voice. "There's no 'dog' in dough…"

4

CHOLOEPUS DIDACTYLUS

Moojag and I fly straight past Phil's Bar and up over the winding path that leads to the woods. The cool evening breeze skims our faces as we zoom in and out of the tall forest trees looking for signs of life. There are no Pofs, and not a single Conqip to be seen, either. They must still be on the Isle of Brix.

"Rest a minute," says Moojag, plopping me down and sitting cross-legged in the sweet-scented dewy grass. It's quiet, save for a single chirping bird. The mousy little wren perches on the rim of Moojag's top hat, before fluttering her speckled wings and quickly taking off again.

"Sweet," I say, smiling as 'Desiree' flies away.

"*Non,*" says Moojag, shaking his head.

"*Non?*"

"Look!" he whispers loudly, pointing to a nearby tree. "Mossy lump." A long-armed animal with wiry brown fur covered in blue-green algae, sporting the widest grin and a chipped tooth, is squatting there in a shallow pit. I glance at Moojag and press a finger to my lips, but the sloth has already spotted us and is glaring back. The poor creature is frozen still. They're stuck in the middle of doing a VERY long poo! "*Choloepus didactylus*," whispers Moojag, slowly edging back to hide behind a tree. "Two-fingered sloth. Only ten left."

I peek back. "I knew they were endangered but only ten left in the world?" I whisper. "Didn't they live in South America? How'd they end up here?"

"Captives, down in Gajoomdom. Like us. All ten of them."

So those Conqips snatched every last living sloth? "Why did they have to have sloths for pets?"

"They just liked making fun, whenever they got bored of bullying Auts and using Pofs. They didn't need much looking after. They survive on just leaves."

That's a long poo for a salad! He must've escaped the Conqips. "What shall we name the poor thing?"

"Marcel, of course."

"Of course?"

"He's delivering a *parcel*, so—"

"Hey—Marcel's twerking!"

Moojag covers his eyes as the sloth shakes his booty, then kicks up the dirt and leaves around him to cover his steaming shipment. Marcel collects an apple lying on the ground beside him and scoops it up in slow motion as though it's a grenade ready to explode. He leans across to dig his other pair of sharp curved claws into the earth and pull himself along the ground with his long, strong arms. We follow his trail out of the woods—very slowly... He might as well be a snail at this pace: each Marcel stretch, a torturous half-step for us.

No less than thirty minutes later, we arrive at the top of Box Hill. The sky has turned a cocktail of oranges, pinks, and reds, with the sun starting to go down. Marcel stands tall on his hind legs (or are they arms, too?) and takes a deep breath before leaping up and diving down over the other side of the hill. We rush across to find him dropping down a perfectly drilled, metal-lined hole in the ground. "What's a massive well doing here?!" I say, gazing down it. It's so deep you can barely see the bottom. "You think it goes anywhere?"

"We must find out," says Moojag, tipping his hat with a bow. I crouch down to lower my feet inside, but Moojag grabs hold of my arms and lifts me up into the air with him before hovering us both down the cold vertical shaft. We land, several metres deep, onto a strangely soft bed of apples, berries, flowers... cracked bird eggs and limp lizards! Is this some sort of sloth feast?

Marcel, about to turn right a few feet ahead, cranes his neck and spots us climbing off the pile. He scrambles, scratching at the curved metal wall as he spins round in circles, then scurries back in our direction in a panic. He tries climbing back up the pipe, but falls flat on his back with his furry arms (and legs?) in the air.

Shhhhhhccccchhhhhhhhhssssccccchhhh!

"What's that?" I ask, looking back down the pipe.

"Water," Moojag answers. Marcel curls up into a ball and squeezes his eyes and mouth firmly shut. I look up the shaft and turn back to find Moojag and Marcel both holding their noses. A stream of water is flowing toward us from the other end of the pipe. I grab hold of Moojag's hand as the water suddenly swells and rushes in. It sweeps us up and carries us fast along the long, straight pipe, round a bend, and then a long *long* way down another one, before lifting us up and spitting us back out onto the ground outside.

Sprawled flat on the floor, we gaze up and look around. Everything looks different.

This is *not* Box Hill.

5

SHENBIE

Marcel shakes his frizzy, soaking wet fur and drags himself very slowly out of the pool of shimmering, algae-coated water. Moojag snaps his hat against his knee, popping it back into shape and making the shivering sloth jump. I wring the water out of my Brix t-shirt as Marcel crawls away. Moojag and I both scan the place.

There are only a few trees dotted around. Withering and leafless. Not full and green like the ones on Box Hill. Just beyond, there's a little lake, and on the other side of it stand two wooden huts guarded by a long, thick, wire fence.

"This is not the Real World, is it?"

Moojag shakes his head. "Over there," he calls,

pointing to the horizon and two buildings poking out of the water. One has a thick, rounded end, like a pickled cucumber; the other's is pointed, like a jagged-edged triangular piece of glass. "The Gherkin," he says, flapping his wings. "It had high-powered lifts that could carry 378 people at once! And Piano's Shard. 309.6 metres. Tallest pre-Surge skyscraper."

"London Tops?"

Moojag nods, shaping a heart with his fingers. "Welcome home."

"Let us not forget the 'Undershaft'," calls a deep voice, out of somewhere. I turn to face an older man. He has white eyebrows, a long pointy moustache, and is wearing a twinkling tangerine PIE.

"Who is he?" I whisper, as the man gives Moojag the thumbs up.

"*Ca c'est oncle* Shenbie," answers Moojag, leaping over to shake his hand. I look round to check for Marcel as Moojag takes a bow, but the sloth has vanished.

"Indeed, Shenbie *c'est moi.* I am an old friend of Monzi's nan."

Moojag shakes his head. "He's Moojag now," I explain. My brother nods.

"I see," says the man with a wink and a nod. "Well, it's surely swell to see you again, Moo...Jag? To see *anyone*, quite frankly." He turns to me. "Would you, by any chance, be little Nem?" I nod as he steps over and takes my hand. "Not so little, now, of course," he says, inspecting my long fingers. "I can see your nan in you," he adds, computing my face. "How *is* that feisty friend of mine? Haven't seen her since you all took off for Surrey Isles."

"Good," I answer. "But she can't seem to remember very much anymore, and not for very long."

"Ah. Well, us oldies might have survived the Surge, but there was no escaping the Big D."

"Big D?"

"Dementia epidemic. In the end, people as young as fifty were affected. Nearly forty percent of the population! The stress of the pre-Surge world, not to mention all the sugar and toxins in the food and water, took a toll on us and prematurely shrunk our brain cells."

"Are you here alone?" I ask, gazing at the huts.

"He is not," says Moojag, waving his hand in my face. No, brother, I mean here in London Tops.

"Pretty much," says Shenbie, biting a nail. "I was one of the few who stayed behind. I could never leave my beloved London."

"Do you know about Gajoomdom?" I ask, screwing up my nose. "And the Conqips?" I whisper, scanning round.

The man grimaces, placing a heavy hand on my shoulder. "We don't talk of *them* here."

"We're in trouble," says Moojag. "They've taken Box Hill!"

"The neurodivergents are being held captive," I explain. "The Conqips have got these huge pipes underground," I add, pointing to the massive metal hole behind us.

"So this is the work of Aldon?" he asks, peering down it.

"Actually, it's Brix."

"Who the devil is Brix. Poor lad." I glare at the man for suggesting that Brix could be even the tiniest bit 'poor'. I do feel a little bit sorry for him, though. "The Conqips are all lost souls. Always controlled by someone, probably had everything done for him. Bound to explode at some point."

"Can you help us?"

"Look," he says, shaking his head, "I would love to

help, of course I would, but this hole is nothing but trouble for London Tops. We've had a bunch of small earthquakes this past week, so I feared the Conqips might be plotting to dig for fuel again. We were all set to fill up the hole with cement!"

"Do not!" wails Moojag, somersaulting over him. "The sloths!"

Shenbie's eyes widen.

"And Kitty," I add.

"I can't cement because of sloths? And who the devil is Kitty?"

"A sloth named Marcel is storing food in the well."

"Silly me. Of course he is."

"No, really, he is," I say.

"Can you not kick the sloth out?"

"*Non.*"

"Well, you're going to have to, I can't risk those selfish men getting their dirty hands on London Tops. Where would you all go when Box Hill is no more? Boat house on the Newcastle Nile? A beach hut atop Ben Nevis? *Hmm?*" He shakes his head. "Suspected not."

"So what are we going to do?" I ask him.

"I'm afraid you're on your own, folks."

I glance back at Moojag and wonder what's behind the blank expression. Probably still processing what Shenbie said. "You are a Conqip!" he exclaims, glaring at the man.

"How *dare* you," shouts Shenbie, hands on hips. "I am no such abominable thing."

"You talk like one," I say, nodding.

"Would rather die than be one of *them*. Why on earth do you think I'm still here?"

"You didn't have the guts to leave?" I blurt. And now I feel like my stomach has turned inside out.

"You'd better both leave, before I fetch that cement we saved for a 'rainy day', and then you end up stuck over here with me. And nobody wants that."

I grab Moojag's hand and pull him back toward the well. "Looks like we will have to sort this out ourselves."

"An 'earthquake day', you mean," Moojag calls over his shoulder. "*Au revoir…*"

6

QIPS AND CONS

Moojag and I plummet the well and glide along its curved bottom. We gaze down the long dark pipe for a moment, before getting on our hands and knees and starting to crawl.

It smells of ripened citrus and metal. The floor feels sticky, and there's something strange on the path ahead of us. A chain of wet leaves and fruit segments, and a strange, muffled rattling sound growing louder. "*Shhh*," I whisper. "It's a sloth trail."

Moojag tuts, dodging some slippery, discarded fruit peel. "*What* trail?"

"It's Marcel," I explain. A few feet ahead of us, all curled up and snoring at the end of the trail, sure enough, is Marcel. "Having a pit stop."

"Mid-way?" says Moojag, raised brow.

"Needs must." Dad said sloths don't have much energy, so he must be busy saving some.

"*My* needs must," declares my brother, charging past me with a huff. The stunned creature yelps as Moojag grabs his slimy arm before swinging back round to grab my not-so-slimy one. He zooms us both all the way to the end of the pipe, then shuttles us over the hoard pile and up out of the well. Marcel screeches as Moojag sets him down and, with his two very long, sharp, curved claws, rips off Moojag's top hat. He scuttles backward and flips over onto his tummy, then stretches his arms out in front to drag himself away. Moojag leaps up and down clasping his head as Marcel makes for the woods, with the hat gathering up leaves and dirt as he goes. Poor sloth must be terrified. We shouldn't really have picked him up, but stay in that pipe and he would have been a truly petrified sloth!

"We'll get the hat back, don't worry," I say. "And we'll clean it up, too."

We rush back to Phil's and tell everyone all about Marcel and the well. When we mention Shenbie, Gran's eyes light up. In fact, her whole body is sparkling a brilliant copper-gold! Where did she find that delicious new PIE skin?

"Darling Shenbie!" she says, as Dad closes the black box beside her. The old 'Emergency PIE' box! Gran's smile drops into a pout and she's quiet for a moment.

"What is it, Nem Avti?"

"My poor old Qip friend ended up all alone."

"He's not on his own," I tell her. "What's a Qip? What happened to him?"

"It all started after the solar and wind plants got torn up by the earthquakes," she explains, looking round at Dad and Phil. "The government, made up of Qips and Cons, wanted to start fracking for oil and gas again." Gran checks Uncle Aldon and shakes her head at him. "Shenbie—a Qip—and I—a Con—joined forces to campaign against it. We won, of course, but the others hated the idea of living naturally. So the Qips ousted him. And I didn't agree with the Cons, so I left them, too. Your uncle was furious, called me a 'traitor'—"

"*Treacherous* traitor," croaks Aldon.

"And then," continues Gran, sneering back at him, "Aldon and co. went and joined forces with the Qips, just to spite me! And that's when the nasty lot became the 'Conqip Group'."

Aldon huffs. "The Great Surge put a stop to any

chance of fracking," he adds. "But we'd already built our super bunker. Living right under your noses, all along—"

Gran laughs at him. "Until the glorious day we found you out!"

"That's when you left?" I ask her. "For Kenya, with Sophia and Stella?"

Gran nods. "We couldn't tell a soul, you understand."

"Why didn't Shenbie come to Box Hill with us?"

"Shenbie isn't neurodivergent."

Wait, why didn't we include him anyway? Wasn't that the whole point of the Real World? So everyone would accept each other and embrace their differences? "So what?"

"Once society finally understood neurodiversity," she explains, "they started including more people with disabilities." I nod. "Well, that was all very good and respectable, but most of them only did it to look good and get more business. Sell more stuff." What? How could they be so selfish? "They didn't truly appreciate us or want to really get to know us or hang out with us." Their loss! "And then some of them found their way onto our apps, pretending to have disabilities. They even faked friendships with us." Lying about being someone's friend? Why would anyone do that? They sound like Conqips!

"It became impossible to trust neurotypicals," explains Dad. "We had a duty to protect Auts with complex or invisible needs. To create a world where only verified neurodivergents would live together."

"Verified?"

"Only someone recommended by another neurodivergent could be accepted into our community."

What? How is *that* okay? "How could you be sure if someone was autistic, or neurodivergent? When they—we—are *all* different?"

"Of course it was harder to tell, because back then Auts had excellent masking skills. They could act just like other people, to fit in. But actually, once you spent a little time with them, especially if you were autistic or ND, you could quickly pick up on all their wonderful traits."

"Like hyperfixation," says Moojag.

"Definitely," says Gran. "Neurodivergents get really into stuff. Hyperfocusing on interests for days, months, even years. Neurotypicals just can't see some things the way we do. Or just *won't*."

"It wasn't foolproof," says Dad, shaking his head,

"but it worked for us, back then."

"Shenbie understood," says Gran. "He could have come, but he stayed behind to support the other London Toppers who refused to leave home."

"What now, Nem Avti?" asks Phil, listening out for Conqips at the door.

"I must go to the old Qip," answers Gran, turning to face the Captain and pulling up her PIE hood, "and request his help."

"We'll come with you," I say, holding out my hand to Moojag. "But I don't think you'll get much help." He nods, swinging me round for the door.

"Take care, kids!" calls Dad, as we fly out after Gran.

7

KITTY IN THE WELL

Peeking out through the trees, we spot a ring of Pofs dancing up on the hill. Dozens of bulging arm muscles throwing long steel rods about like spears.

"Pof constructors," whispers Moojag, as the tiny tutu-wearing bodybuilders with wings trail off in a straight line down the hill and out of sight. Before I can speak, my brother hovers off after them.

"Come," says Gran, patting her back and bending over. "*PIE Fly*!"

I climb on and we speed off after Moojag, but we don't get very far when he stalls to turn around and shoo us back. "Brix!" he whispers, landing with a wobble. We all lay flat on the ground and peer over the hill. Brix is directing a group of Pofs building a metal tower over two floors. Orange Pof is perched on the lower level, twinkly legs dangled over the side. She dissects a brown ball in the palm of her hand (the chocolate orange?) into segments, keeping a beady eye on her fellow workers, then pops a piece into her mouth. She nods, grinning.

"We'll get enough oil," Brix bellows over the churning cement truck parked beside the tower, "to live off for the rest of our lives."

"Those divergent mutes," declares a drunken Travis, lurching behind him, "won't get a drop!" Brix's glass tips as he does a celebratory jig and the champagne splashes across Travis' black dinner jacket.

He huffs, but Brix just steps back and slaps him on the forehead. "Look what you made me do, now, Quiffy."

I shake my head. Why would they want oil, anyway? We don't need any. Nobody does. Brix orders the Pofs about some more, then struts off for the woods with Travis grovelling behind. Moojag bolts up to sit cross-legged and shuts his eyes. Gran and I turn to face the trees. "What's that?" she asks, pointing to a small, greenish-brown figure stepping out. It's a small Pof wearing a flower and leaf-covered tutu. She topples over trying to hover up, weighed down by a bulging sack, wings buckling at her sides.

"It's Kitty," says Moojag, as the little Might swings the big bag over her shoulder, skips out, and hovers straight past us, before finally zooming up the hill.

Must be some really good stuff in there, not to notice us. We follow her to the other side and watch her drop the bag down the well before jumping in after it. "That's the way," I say, "to London Tops!"

Gran creeps forward and peers down into the shaft. "I see fruits and flowers… and eggs? Quite a hoard—"

"Who's there!" Kitty's voice echoes back up.

Gran leaps away from the well and pokes herself to activate PIE's Invisibility Function. "Going in," says her legless body as she quickly disappears on the spot. "Grab Kitty when she gets out, and take her back with you!" We nod to the rustling pile of leaves, before Gran finally drops down the well with a whoosh.

"*Oooouch...*" screams Kitty. "Off my stuff!"

The Pof catapults back out, clutching an empty sack. She pauses to wipe her lips then scrunches up her nose and huffs at Moojag and I. "Why you not lock up?" she asks, scanning us both.

"We managed to escape. To come to find you!" I

explain.

Moojag steps over and puts an arm around her shoulders. "Come back, Kitty, we need your help."

"No," she says, crossing her arms tightly. "I live in *there* now." She points her little finger in the direction of the woods. "No one find me," she adds, shimmying her busy skirt. "Me made it! Leaves, flowers, sticky stuff—"

"Camouflage?" I ask.

"Not camel fudge!" she answers, shaking her head. "Sloth!"

"Are you a sloth now?" asks Moojag.

Kitty smiles, nodding. "My new family," she answers, waving goodbye before whizzing off back to the woods.

"*Hellooooo*, goodbye, little girl?" calls a thrilled, Scottish man's voice coming from right behind us. Wats? We swivel round. Moojag bows and I curtsey. Only Wats-knows-why.

"Where did you come from!" I say, mirroring Wats' outstretched arms.

"Would you believe there's a magical mystery tunnel, all the way from Juniper to this, here, very Box Hill!"

How is there suddenly a tunnel that no one ever thought to mention before! "There is?" I ask, frowning hard.

"Indeed. We came together!" he says, leaping aside to reveal the two shrinking Peace Gajooms behind him. "The little ones must have smelled something pungent, because they bolted right away and led me to a hole in the ground—the hole that led to the tunnel—this very tunnel we followed all the way here!" He does one of his little jigs and finally stands victorious, poised as a statue but with arms still stuck in the air.

"That one?" I ask, pointing to the well.

"Er," he mutters, spinning round, "nope, *thatta* one." He skips over to a wooden hatch surrounded by a mound of moss and leaves. "We've been all *across the universe*, don't you know, to get back! Get back! *Get baaaaack...*" The mini white Gajooms bounce on after him and stick themselves firmly down either side of the hatch, before bending over to form an arch.

"You found the secret passage, then," says Moojag, tapping his nose.

Why didn't my brother just tell us about this when he found us here? "Why didn't you send *us* all 'across the universe' to Gajoomdom, in the first place?!"

"Too risky," says Moojag, scanning round. "It's the Conqips' way in and out. And, by the way, they were always in and out on those poor candy robots!"

"Gondolas and magical mystery tours are so much more fun," says Wats, skipping around me and beckoning the Gajooms to his side.

"So that's how they've been stealing our tech and food!" Moojag nods. "How they must've gotten here before us, after the… bomb," I whisper.

"They've got the Pofs building something," Moojag informs Wats.

"That metal well," I explain, "and a giant pipe all the way to London Tops!"

"And that tower over there—" adds Moojag, pointing to it.

"No one's gonna change our world, baby." Wats marches around us beating his air drum and shaking his head.

"What *is* that thing they're building?" I ask.

"Just a rumour," whispers Wats as he leans in close, "but Brix is fracking. No good."

"We know he's no good," huffs Moojag, arms

crossed.

"I mean—he's drilling underground to get gas and oil," Wats says, spinning around. "They'll flush the well with water, sand, and acid, to create great big cracks in the rock and pump out all the good stuff for fuel!"

"And keep living their selfish lives... *here*," I add, "now that they've hunted nearly all the animals and stolen our veg!"

"Here, there, and everywhere," declares Wats.

"Oh no, they won't," I say, turning away.

8

CEMENT OR BERRIES?

"Here I come!" calls Gran's echo.

We all jump back from the well as she bounds out like a Gajoom. She lands headfirst with a bounce, protected by her puffed-up hood, then bolts upright and shakes all our hands in turn. The luminous silver-and-white-striped Peace Gajooms leap over and bump their sugary selves up against her leg. She pats their heads (or their bottoms—who knows which way up is up) and smiles.

"Who are you, girl?" she asks, stroking the entire side of my face. "Do I know you?"

"You do. I'm Nema."

She turns away for three long seconds, then swings back and grabs my shoulder. "Of course you are! But why are you here?"

"I—"

"Not important," she says. "I've seen Shenbie!"

"Is he going to help?"

"YES!" she says, scooping up the Gajooms and swinging round with them tucked inside her arms.

"How?" asks Moojag.

Gran squints at us and cocks her head. "Pardon?"

"What's Shenbie going to do?" asks Wats.

"Do you know," she says, standing perfectly still, "I haven't the foggiest!" She giggles, dropping the Gajooms. They just roll over and wobble, bouncing back up. Gran must be forgetting again. "There *is* a plan!" she says, gazing at our poised, hopeful faces. "I simply can't recall *what*."

"You gotta think for yourself, woman—" cries Wats.

"Try retracing your steps," I say. "You went down the tunnel to London Tops, then what?"

"That's right!" she says, wide-eyed. "I found my dear friend Shenbie waiting on the other side." I nod and take her hand. She squeezes it and bites her lip. "He's going to fill the hole with... cement? Or was it berries? Cherries? Or, he *wasn't*..." Wow, she's actually forgotten everything.

"OH, don't be so nosey, all of you," she says, fuming. "What do you want from me? Who *are* you all, anyway!"

"Hold your horses, Lady Madonna," chants Wats, skipping away from her. "It'll come back to you. All in good time. Unlike my sense of smell, of course. Oh no, not at any time at all! Don't ask me why. I asked Dr Robert. No reply. A real nowhere man..." Is Wats still talking to *us*, or is he only lost in his merry land of song titles? "You ain't seen me, right!" he declares, tapping his nose and scanning the place, before leaping back down the tunnel with the springy Peace Gajooms in tow.

"We better get back to the hut," I say, "until Gran remembers again." I glance at her peering wrinkly face. "Back to your Jack, Gran?" She shrugs her shoulders. "After you, Moojag."

"Then back for Kitty, *oui*," he says. "And my hat," he adds, tapping his head. I nod. Gran lets me climb onto her back and we head for the pier.

Leaving Gran there, safe with Dad, we sneak out at dusk to go on our Kitty/sloth hunt through the woods. We don't find her, or any sloths, but then Moojag spots some scattered leaves and berries. "We're getting close," he says, leaping over the fallen fruit. The trail leads us out of the woods, all the way back to the metal well. "She must have gone down again," he says, shaking his head. I peer inside. The tip of an iridescent wing and a little round behind are sticking up out of the feast. Kitty's face is buried in the pile, too busy munching to notice.

"Hey!" calls Moojag. She jumps, startled, and rolls off to reveal a top hat-wearing Marcel, tummy-side-up and clutching a pink-iced doughnut.

"Busy now!" she calls, staring up googly-eyed, before turning back to nuzzle the hoard. "Go! Brix comin—"

"Did he throw you in there?" Moojag whispers loudly, but she doesn't answer.

We drop down, but she wrestles us and kicks the feast, sending everything flying up around the well.

Shhhhhhccccchhhhhhhhsssscccchhhh...

Here we go again!

Moojag clutches Marcel's foot and grabs Kitty's bicep with his other hand. "Brix threw me in," she cries, as the water comes rushing toward us. "Slomo not let me go!"

The water floods in, flushing us all the way back through the pipe and up out onto London Tops.

9

GUMP'S BABY

"You again?" says Shenbie, as we pick ourselves up. "We weren't expecting you back. What happened to Nem Avti?"

"Gran couldn't remember your plan," I say, shaking off the water.

"Well, *this* wasn't it," he says, inspecting the two slimy creatures slumped beside us.

"We were looking for this one," explains Moojag, pointing at Kitty sat drenched and cross-legged on the floor, "and got swept up here again."

"So this is the sloth?" he asks, bending down beside trembling Marcel. "Now, what are you doing in a well?" he asks him. "In the English Isles, no less!"

"*Marcel*," explains Moojag, "was a Conqip pet."

"Enough faffing about," says Shenbie. "Now,

listen. The next time this thing flushes, it could be hydrochloric acid." My brother's eyes widen. "And you may not make it back out looking the same way you did when you went in."

"HCl—hydrogen and chlorine dissolved in water," declares Moojag, raised brow. "Breathed in or swallowed causes oedema, spasm, asphyxia, chemical pneumonia, acidosis, haemolysis, renal failure, DEATH." WHAT? How does my brother know so much about this HCl stuff!

"It'll burn your skin first," warns Shenbie, "before it does all that. You'll have to stay put; pray she remembers before it's too late."

"We can't just wait and do nothing," I say. "What *was* your plan?"

"Mission Vitriolage," he says. "The emergency PIE withstands any chemical. Nem Avti was going to find the Conqip, coax him back to the pipe and into the acid. No Conqip leader, no fracking, end of."

Brix is nasty, but he doesn't deserve an acid attack! No one does. I should've taken Gran's emergency PIE. But there has to be another way. "Why don't we just go back and get rid of the acid, and all the fracking stuff?"

Shenbie stands back holding his hands in prayer.

"Out of the question!—"

"Look after Marcel and Kitty," I say, turning to grab Moojag's wing and jumping on his back. "We're going home." But Kitty scoops up Marcel and wraps his long arms around her belly. She prepares to leap down the well before us, but as she steps over the edge, the ground begins to tremble and cracks start appearing all round the well.

"Get back!" calls Shenbie, before a swooping, swirling sound echoes out from the big hole. "Second thoughts," he shouts. "RUN!"

A giant, winding, column-shaped wave rises up and tosses a sizzling sloth onto the floor beside us. The wave collapses, splashing all over the ground around the well. Shenbie rips off his glowing, tangerine PIE skin to cover the frazzled animal. "To fresh water!" he calls, crouching down in only a pair of white shorts with the London Underground map printed on them. He scoops her up and sprints to the pond. Now we truly are stuck over here, if this is the hydrochloric acid Shenbie was on about.

Marcel rolls up his innocent, glazed-over eyes at us as Moojag grabs his left arm and I gently take hold of his right. We haul him up and chase after Shenbie and the new sloth.

The soaked creature at Shenbie's feet whimpers at Marcel as we plop him down beside her. He scratches at her wet fur with his long claws, combing it in all directions. Is she smiling, or is that her daily sloth grin? Whichever way, she doesn't seem hurt by the acid.

"Perhaps," says Shenbie, "it was sufficiently diluted?"

"Symbiotic shield!" exclaims Moojag, scanning the wiry, wet fur of the sloth's slimy long arm. It looks as though it's covered in green and yellow highlights. "Enzyme-producing algae and microbes. Cancels out the acid," he says, swiping a sample of the luminous goo with the tip of his finger. "*Gump.*"

"Gump?"

"For 'gumption'. Brave and resilient, like elastic—always bouncing back."

Does Moojag know this sweet sloth? Or are all sloths this way?

Gump lets out a tiny high-pitched cry that sounds like a human baby calling for its mother, then her arms swing out as if begging for a hug. I step forward to stroke her, but she wriggles away. Has Marcel's grimace turned slightly downward? Is this what a *fearful* sloth grin looks like? What has Gump said?

"Lost baby," explains Moojag. "Conqip attack." Marcel's whole body jolts, as though he understood my brother's words, and he buries his head in the crook of Gump's arm. Has a Conqip taken her baby? Gump swipes her claws across the crown of her head, slicking back the fur. With it pulled back so tight, she almost looks bald.

Wait! Bald? Brix! "Brix?!" I call, nodding at the sloth. She shrieks and squeezes her eyes shut. "He took her baby?" I ask, turning to Moojag. "Then threw her down the well?" Moojag nods.

"Despicable, sloth-hungry brutes," shouts Shenbie, charging off. "That is the last straw! I'll be back," he yells, already halfway around the pond.

What if the Conqips weren't just keeping those poor sloths alive as pets, but actually saving them as emergency food?

Shenbie runs into one of the huts, leaving the door swinging wide open. A person peers out and disappears back inside, spotting us. So he isn't alone, after all. Shenbie leaps back out in his PIE again. Better. And carries a great big bundle. He lugs it over, plants it down, and releases two wide rainbow straps to reveal a huge pile of glowing multi-coloured material. "The original Emergency PIE prototype," he announces. "Entrusted to me by your Gran—for a rainy day." Moojag looks up to the sky. Clear blue, not a cloud in sight. "Or, rather, a *hydrochloric acid* day," adds Shenbie, with a wink. Hmm, who doesn't love a hydrochloric acid day… "Now then," he adds, stepping to my side, "I think we could rustle up an acid-proof vessel from this old gear. What do you say?"

Moojag does a somersault over the pile to shake his hand. I've never made a vessel—how would I know? Apparently my brother does, though. He knew enough to make the Gajooms. Pulling out the material created by Dad, Mum, and Gran so many years ago, Moojag hovers up until the whole length of it hangs in the air. "Needs a charge," he says, eyeing up its lifeless hexagonal skin cells.

"It can have all of *my* juice," says Shenbie, detaching the Spondylux shell from his chest and switching it with the one attached to the material. He crosses his fingers and starts to pace up and down, whilst Moojag sits cross-legged and I clasp my hands.

Finally, a single cell lights up. Then another. And another, until each and every one is twinkling bright.

Shenbie voices "*Reset*" into Spondylux, and the material stops flashing before turning a uniform, sparkling copper-gold colour. Just like the PIE Gran's wearing now.

Moojag lays it down flat on the ground. "*Dished bottom,*" he calls into Spondylux; then, "*Self-sealing sides.*"

"Very good," says Shenbie. "When you land, you just call 'surface', to release the seal. Take care not to get spotted—the Conqips won't be far away now that the flushing has begun."

With our emergency PIE vehicle ready to go, we pile in and Shenbie calls '*Sub*!'. We wait silently, with only Marcel and Gump's chattering teeth to distract us, as we're sealed inside the vessel. Then Shenbie plunges us down with the next flush, in a golden submarine that Wats would be proud of!

10

SLOTH HUNT

"*IF*," Moojag calls into Spondylux as we cruise up to the well at the other end. The Invisibility Function. Good, so no one will see us coming.

We fly out with the wave and glide a few metres along the ground. I listen out for bullies then whisper, "*Surface*," into Spondylux. The submarine's sides release and we crawl out. Moojag hauls up Marcel and Gump, as Kitty throws me over her shoulder, and they fly us straight to the forest edge.

Kitty tips me off her wing and hovers after Moojag to escort the sloths up onto a high tree branch. I crane my neck and wave goodbye. They must be relieved to be home, but, hanging upside down, their grins now look like frowns.

A rustling whispers through the leaves and twigs

on the ground. I quickly jump behind the tree beside me.

"Do you smell sloth?" shouts an angry man's voice. Moojag hovers up higher but brushes Marcel's arm, giving the poor creature a fright. The sloth loses his grip on the branch and drops all the way down to the forest floor with a thump. These creatures might be slow and a bit clumsy, but they can survive a 100-foot fall without a single injury. Marcel's all right!

"It's raining sloths, B'!" cries Travis, belly swaying as he bounces up and down.

"How delightfully convenient," says Brix, with a smarmy grin. "Hasn't landed in its poo again, has it?" he adds, glancing away. Travis steps cautiously up to Marcel and probes the ground around him. Brix peeks back, wincing. "*Ugghh*, are you stupid?!" He pokes Travis out of the way. "Of course you are!"

"It's Bogey Face!" says Travis, hands clasped.

"About time we roasted the old toad, before he gets too gamey."

"Oh yes!" says Travis, nodding, as drool dribbles from the corner of his mouth. "While he's still nice and juicy." They don't really mean to *eat* Marcel, do they? How can they be thinking about eating their own pet, let alone a wild animal!

"TRAVIS," hollers Brix, snapping his fingers in the man's face and making him jolt. "Don't just stand there," he says, wafting his hand over Marcel. "Take Slomo to the Old Fort. Have the men hunt down the rest for the chop, too. We'll need copious amounts of finger-licking fried limbs for our fracking celebration party." What?! Fried! I hold my hand over my mouth and gag.

Travis bows his head. "Yes, *master*."

"Don't be so facetious, Travis. Does not suit you."

Ooooo, good one! What does *that* mean? *Facetious, facetious, facetious*. Maybe he's particular about his shoes? Brix and Travis waltz off, dragging Marcel behind them by the claws. I look away. We're not letting those nasties eat him! Not ANY of them.

I call to my brother and he hovers down, shaking his head. "We have to figure out a way to stop them," I say "before it's too late!" Without a word, or even a somersault, Moojag throws me over his shoulder and flies us back to the floating hut.

We creep up to the door and tap twice.

"Who's there," whispers Dad.

"Us," I answer.

"Nem?"

"Yes. Quick—open up!"

He releases the door. Mum is stood there beside him with arms open wide. She scoops us in and squeezes us tight. "We were worried!" I would've thought you'd be used to us disappearing by now, Mum. "What happened?"

"Got flushed," answers Moojag. "Hydrochloric acid."

Mum's eyes widen and she starts to pat us down. "Are you hurt?"

"We're fine," I say, presenting the rolled-up PIE submarine.

Dad steps closer and strokes its golden cells. "Our prototype material," he says, nodding to Mum.

"Shenbie had it. We turned it into an acid-proof vessel."

"Ingenious," he says, clasping my shoulder with his heavy hand. I pat Moojag's. Moojag pokes Mum's.

Uncle Aldon grunts. "I suspect the boys have run out of meat," he says, pouting. "Blockhead Brix started fracking again, has he?"

"Yes," I answer. "And he's snatching baby sloths, too! They're hunting them all right now and holding them at the Old Fort. They're planning to fry them for their 'fracking feast celebration'!"

"Marcel for starters," adds Moojag. *Ugghh. Literally.*

"That lazybones is well past his consume-by date," says Aldon. *Ugghh.* "Baby sloth, though," he adds, "yum yum..." *Eww. NO.*

"That's enough swearing, now, brother," says Gran, sealing Aldon's mouth with the cupped palm of her wrinkly hand. "Sick, greedy Conqips at their old tricks again." She jogs over to us and swipes the PIE vessel from Dad. "Wasn't enough to exterminate all the animals on Juniper—now they're resorting to their own pets to fill their guts?" She cloaks herself with the PIE, wrapping it around her shoulders. "The plan!" she cries.

"Where are you going, Nem Avti?" I call after her as she marches for the door.

"To Shenbie. We have to stop this!"

"You remembered your plan?"

"Of course I remember," she says, cocking her head and letting out a little chuckle. "Me—forget a plan?!"

"Well," hollers Moojag, "what is it, then?"

"Time for a taste of his own medicine." Aldon

winces at Gran's words and curls back up into a ball. He's already had a taste of *his* own medicine.

"But the plan's changed," I say, leaping over to grab her arm. "No one is going to kill *anyone*."

"Then what do you suppose we do, girl?"

"First, we need to get rid of that fracking tower."

Gran looks me up and back down at my bare legs peeking out from the ridiculous, oversized Brix t-shirt. "Ha!"

"What will become of the sloths!" says Moojag, frowning hard.

"He's right," says Dad.

"Have you forgotten," says Captain Phil, leaning in, "about all the Auts next door?"

Adam and Izzy! Sophia and Stella!

"Of course not," says Dad. "But we've tried getting them out—"

"We need a Conqip," says Phil, "to open all those locks. It's our only hope of getting in."

Moojag shuffles up to them. "You could get one to talk about their special interest," he says, leaning in. "You'll have enough time to sneak everyone out, all at once."

"Great idea," agrees Dad, turning to Phil. "Captain, you go to the Auts and come up with the diversion plan, okay? Meanwhile, the kids and I will go rescue these sloths." He turns back to Gran. "Mum," he says, placing his hand on her shoulder, "can you find your own way back to Shenbie?" Gran tuts at him and crosses her arms. "Well, your emergency PIE can protect you from the acid," he reassures her, taking back the deflated submarine, "so you won't get hurt." He turns to me. "You and Monzi will keep hold of this for now."

Moojag shakes his head, frowning so hard that his brows meet in the middle. "*Moojag*," he says, cross-armed.

"Once the sloths are rescued and hidden somewhere safe, we'll get straight to Gran and Shenbie and put a stop to this fracking."

Moojag bows and I nod, as Aldon tries picking himself up off the floor. "Take me with you," he says, hobbling, "I could be *your* distraction." Does Uncle really want to help, or is he up to his old tricks? I frown, looking round at my brother.

"Only if he is not rude," says Moojag, arms crossed.

Aldon sniffs, placing a hand to his chest. "*Moi?*"

he says, with a snort. “That’s an Aut’s job.”

Moojag huffs, turning for the door. I glare back at the hunched Conqip. “You didn’t mean that, did you, Uncle?” He shakes his head. “Bye, then,” I tell him and wave to the others. “We’ll be back soon!”

“Don’t worry, my loves,” answers Mum, turning to Phil. “We’ll make sure all the Auts get out safe. Won’t we?” Phil nods, stepping forward to hug me with a single buff arm. He swings out his other one for Moojag. My brother leans in quickly, but then leaps right away.

Dad opens the door and peeks out. “All clear,” he says, waving us through first. It’s darker now, with the sun almost down, and there’s a nip in the air. “Right,” says Dad, sneaking out and marching on ahead with his arm raised like a pre-Surge tour guide, “to the Old Fort!”

I leap in front of him. “Moojag can get us there in a flash.” He frowns, looking at Moojag’s fluttering wings; beautiful iridescent cells glimmering in the early evening light.

“Both of us?”

“Climb on,” I say, pushing down on a wing. “They’re super strong. They won’t break.”

“I should hope *not*,” says Dad, carefully hopping

onto Moojag's back and gently gripping his wing.

"*You* won't break, either," I say, jumping on, as Moojag hovers off the ground then swoops us over Zig Zag Path to the old Military Road.

11

OLD FORT KITCHEN

"Approaching LDS!" calls Moojag, pointing to the Old Fort now in clear sight. "London Defence Scheme," he adds. He looks pleased with himself. "Built to protect London from continental invaders."

"Very true, son," says Dad, head tilted and with the hint of a smile. "Abandoned shortly after, in 1906."

"That is correct, Jack," nods Moojag. "Well done."

"Watch out for Major Labelliere!" calls Dad, as we speed past the grave of a local legend.

"Gran said he's one of our ancestors?" I call, glimpsing the words etched into the headstone.

...Eccentric resident of Dorking,

buried here head downwards 1800

"Yep. Interesting fellow. Left two peculiar wishes

in his will: for the children of his landlord to dance on his coffin, and to be buried here upside-down!"

"Why?"

"Well, he fell in love with a woman," explains Dad, "who didn't love him back. His lonely heart just couldn't take it and then he lost his mind, too."

"But why headfirst?"

"Because he thought the world was going 'topsy-turvy'. So, by being buried upside-down, he would eventually 'end up the right way around'."

Hmm. So would that make him the right way up again by now?

"*Bah*," says Moojag, with a huff. "Buried coffins do not turn underground!"

"Well," says Dad, smiling, "I suppose he didn't mean it literally."

"Ugh. *Mon Dieu*."

I pat Moojag's shoulder. "I should like to be buried on a bed of flowers."

"If you were any kind of important in the Middle Ages," he says, grinning back widely, "you might be buried on a feather and wool-stuffed mattress."

"Poor man was truly troubled," says Dad, as

Moojag drops us down in front of the fort's outer stone wall. "They said he predicted the date of his own death..."

We tip-toe after Moojag, along the grass-covered roof of the fort, past the two rows of little metal-hooded chimneys... *Two, Four, Six, Eight, Ten.*

I peek round the corner to the grilled steel gate entrance. The rusty red doors are covered in glossy, dark green ivy. Lime-coloured fuzzy moss has sprouted through the gaps. Wait, that moss is moving! The fuzzy green growth pushes out between the bars and unfurls into a long arm with two claws sticking out its end. Not moss... Marcel! Moojag jolts back, bumping into me. I press a finger to my lips as we step up to the gate and peer through the bars. The rest of the sloths are lined up in cages on a counter. On the opposite side, a giant saucepan of splattering, bubbling liquid on an old stove oven. Oil!

"This thing is bolted from the inside, kids." *When* will he stop saying that! I'm thirteen, for goodness' sake! "Are the sloths trained?" he asks Moojag.

My brother squints, scrunching up his mouth and tapping his chin. "*Oui*," he answers, finally. "But you will need a sloth snack."

Hmm, well, he's a folivore—he eats mostly leaves.

I gaze round, looking for something edible. Right beside us there's a small fig tree. "One of these do?" I ask, picking off a five-lobed leaf.

Moojag nods. "*Ficus carica.* Nutty favorite!"

"Perfect," whispers Dad. "Now, what to do with it?"

Moojag snatches the leaf and leaps over to the gate in one long stride. Marcel's arm shrinks back inside as Moojag waves the leaf back and forth in front of the lock. "We used to play this in Gajoomdom," he says, nodding at Marcel. "When *they* weren't looking." The sloth hooks his claws into the lock and slides it across.

Clunk!

The gate opens and Marcel falls to the ground at Dad's feet. He grabs my ankle, trembling. "It's okay, Marcel," I say, petting his wiry arm. Crusty and moist all at once. Moojag crouches down and nods in Marcel's face, their short, round, upturned noses almost touching.

"Aldon brought them to London Tops," explains Dad, "to study their behaviour. He discovered they had some similar traits to us," he adds, smiling. My brother looks at him, brows drawing closer. Dad places a hand on his shoulder. "Just like them, we are gentle and calm, thoughtful and generous. Clear-sighted and sensible, too."

A thudding sound echoes through the fort walls. "This way," Moojag whispers. "B's back!" He scoops up Marcel and ushers us over to the arch. We sneak out and hide behind a big box-shaped evergreen hedge.

"Why is this gate unlocked, Travis!" The rusty metal gate squeaks and goes *clink* as Brix's voice fades away.

Dad taps my shoulder. "Time for a little Conqip lock-in?!"

"But the sloths..?" I say, glaring back up at him.

"We'll come back for them later."

"What if they *cook* them before we get back!"

"They won't," says Moojag. "Conqip leaders never kill their own prey. And they don't 'partake of *raw* flesh'." *Ewwww*.

"Wait here," Dad tells Moojag. I nod and rush back down through the arch with him to the fort. He grabs the grill, pulling it shut, and I slide the lock closed.

"But they can just unlock it, Dad. Can't they?"

"Sure. That's why we need *that*." He points to a long metal pole resting in the long grass. "Grab the other end!" he whispers, lifting it up. We lean it against the wall beside the doorway and Dad carefully closes in the heavy steel shutters on either side. The rusty hinges squeak as the doors clank together. A yell echoes from the inside. Dad dives for the pole and leans it diagonally, into the top right corner of the doorway. He pushes the other end into the bottom left, wedging it in.

"Not on!" calls a muffled voice. "Open up, this minute!"

Dad dusts off his hands. "This ought to hold 'em for a while," he says, with a wink. I give him a thumbs up and turn to grab a fig branch crammed with coconut- and vanilla-smelling fig leaves, before we race back up to Moojag and Marcel.

12

BACK TO FRACK

"You're safe now," I say, peering round the hedge. Our sloth friend is clung to Moojag's coat, snoring away.

"We can't take him back to the woods," says Moojag. Marcel's eyelids flutter as he tries cocking his head and then nods back off to sleep.

"We'll have to take him with us," says Dad. Moojag nods. "We'll find a nice tree for him at London Tops." Moojag shakes his head and so do I. "No?"

"Only one tree with anything on it where we're going, Dad. What if he doesn't like *that* one?"

A bat swoops in and takes a wide turn, rowing its wings with all its might to fly straight back up into the trees. "I'm sure he'll love it," says Dad. "Two-fingered sloths aren't so fussy about their greens." He does seem to love flowers and insects, too, so he should be just fine.

We join the path down to the well, where Dad unravels our PIE vessel and waits for us all to climb in. There's just enough room for everyone, with Marcel curled up on my lap. I hold still, so as not to disturb his evening snooze and give him a chance to recharge his sloth batteries. Dad shoves us closer to the edge of the hole and jumps in as Moojag calls, "*Seal.*"

We drop down the shaft, landing softly at the bottom. Sixty sloth snores later, and we are underway with the next flush through the pipe, and back out onto dry land in London Tops after thirty more.

"*Surface,*" calls a woman's muffled voice. The vessel peels itself open and a flash of light beams down on us from Gran's glowing PIE skin. Marcel burrows into my arm as I also duck my head out of the glare. "Welcome home, Jack," she says, pulling Dad out. "You've brought friends," she says, squinting at us.

"It's me, Gran," I say, crawling out with Marcel clung to my waist.

"You don't look like Gran."

"Not *your* Gran. *My* Gran." I glance round at Moojag tipping his hat to her.

"Monzi?"

Moojag nods with a sigh.

"*Moojag*," I say.

"Ah yes," Gran replies, with a wink, "and your sister, Nema?" And she's back.

"Where's Shenbie?" asks Dad.

"Hmm. Let's see. Shenbie. Yes, that's right! How did you know?" she says, gazing round. "He, *er*, he went to fetch supplies."

"Of?"

"Cherries?"

Dad looks at us and pouts. Must be wondering why Shenbie would be bringing supplies of cherries. Marcel's nose twitches and he topples to the ground beside the branch of bright green fig leaves.

"There he is!" she says, pointing to a man jogging back round the lake. It's Shenbie with a bag slung across his chest, in only a cowboy hat and his London Underground shorts.

"Here I come, Nem Avti!" he calls, slumped over and gasping for air. They don't get much exercise here, then.

"What's in the bag?" I ask, as he strides over.

"A few provisions!" he answers. "Jack, is that you, boy?" Dad nods, holding out his hand to shake Shenbie's.

Gran leans in to her friend and whispers in his ear, "Did you bring the cement, Man?"

"Cement?" he asks, gazing round at me and Moojag. "And who are these two?"

I glance at my brother. He rocks his head. Of course, the man probably has dementia too, so he's forgotten the 'fill up the well with cement' plan.

"We're going to stop the Conqip from destroying the Real World! Are you with us, Uncle Shenbie?"

He glares at me, then breaks a smile. "Nema?"

"Yep," I say, nodding. "And my brother, Moojag."

"He looks devilishly like little Monzi." Moojag bows. Shenbie cocks his head and breaks another smile. "So what's the plan of attack?" he asks, turning to Gran.

"I say, we swoop in, throw 'em all in the Old Fort and lose the key."

"I say," I say, "we rescue the sloths first, before they get fried!"

"We'll be needing more troops," says Dad. I nod.

"Super Pofs," declares Moojag. Right. We're going to need those last pesky Pofs on side to have any hope of stopping Brix and his men.

"They have the muscle superpower to stop all the drilling and take down the tower."

Dad steps forward and points to Shenbie's bag. "What have you got to offer the Pofs?"

"We have plenty!" he says, pointing to a big, lonesome orange tree. Where did that spring from! Marcel is there, hanging from a low branch, ogling the fruit.

"Perfect," says Moojag, doing a somersault. Right—because a certain Pof would do anything for an actual orange!

"Orange Pof will take down the tower in a second."

"Great. We should split up," says Dad.

I nod to Moojag. "We'll work on the Pofs."

"Good, good. So, Nem Avti, Shenbie—we three will see to Brix," he says, poking Gran. "And Aldon will help us."

Shenbie grunts, taking a step back. "Why would that mean man ever do anything for us?"

"If he's still on our side, he will—" I say, before Dad leaps in and gives the old London Topper the rundown, so I don't have to.

I skip over to the tree, and pull on a branch to pluck

off some oranges. I hand one to Marcel. He reaches out and punches his claw straight through the middle of the fruit, then lifts it above his cocked head to catch the juice drippings in his mouth. "Is it safe to leave him here?"

Shenbie nods. "The London Toppers will take good care of the slimy little geezer." He taps his chin and glances back at Gran. "But wait, what the devil is a sloth doing in the English Isles?"

"A dirty deal with Colombia," she answers. "Conqips got the very last ten endangered sloths. Pets for their underground bunker." If we don't get a move on, they won't be pets for much longer.

Dad shakes his head. "Right," he says, "we meet back at the dock. Hopefully Zoe and Phil will have set the Auts free, and together we can finally stop these nasty Conqips."

I wave goodbye to Marcel, as Shenbie detaches him from the tree and carries him off around the lake. He'll be all right. He's used to humans. And we'll be back for him soon enough.

13

WHAT A WASTE!

Dad, Gran, and Shenbie disappear over the hill for the Fort, cloaked in the soft evening light, as Moojag and I make for the half-built fracking tower.

Orange Pof is still sat on level one, legs dangling. "Aut-Pof," she squeals, squinting at Moojag, "is that you, Silent Boy?" She hovers down in front of us and stares up and down at my bare legs. "Lizard girl lost her skin?" She strokes her sparkling tango-coloured arm, and looks back up smiling. "I have one now!"

"Suits you."

Moojag tuts, hovering up onto the tower. "You have to dismantle, Pof."

"Huh?"

"It's got to go," I add, pretending to punch the steel

pole. "We'll lose Box Hill forever if the Conqips get the oil. And they've done quite enough damage already."

"But my giant chocolate orange!" cries Pof, flying back to Moojag's side.

I rock my head. "There is no giant chocolate orange."

The winged girl's nose wrinkles up as she curls her lip at me. "Lying!" she calls, bumping Moojag.

"Sister doesn't lie," he whispers, arms crossed. "Can't."

"I did bring you this, though!" I call up. The furrowed-brow Pof drops back down and snatches the orange from my hand.

"Is this—" I nod. Cupping the fruit in her hands, Orange Pof gives it a sniff, pokes the dimpled skin then puckers her lips before kissing it softly. She gazes up at me with a grin.

"So you'll help us take down the tower?"

"*Hmm...* All right," she mumbles, "but I'll need more! A LOT more."

"There's a tree-full in London Tops—"

Orange Pof leaps round to the back of the tower and orders the other Pofs to pull it all down. She grabs one of the metal bars connecting the two levels, pulls it out, and snaps it in two over her bulging thigh. The others do the same with each of the other corners, and we all sprint back to the well hole as the whole structure collapses like falling Jenga behind us. “Mission complete,” yells Orange Pof, shaking her head. “Don’t tell Brix Darling!”

“Don’t worry, dear Pof—Brix is at the Fort.”

She shakes her head and swivels around, pointing to a huge hose running across the hill and over the other side. “He’s dumping the waste water into Mole River.”

I swing my arm out to Moojag. “We have to stop him, before he pollutes all the fresh water!” My brother nods and we take off, following the path of the pipe.

“Hey,” Orange Pof calls after us. “Why’s he got that mouldy Gump with him?”

Was Dad too late? How did Brix break down our barricade? Why would he pollute his own water?

“They don’t need water,” declares Moojag, reading my mind. “They only drink champagne. They don’t care if the water gets polluted.”

“What about *us*?” And surely their bubbles are going to run out at some point?

"*What*," answers Moojag, setting us down softly on the bridge crossing the river. "He doesn't need Box Hill. He has *other* islands."

Downstream, two Pofs come through the trees lugging the massive hose toward the river. We crouch down to hide as Brix steps out of the bushes and zips up his trousers. "Get a move on, my little Poffettes," he shouts, plucking Gump off of a branch, as they heave the hose into the water. "We have a celebration feast to prepare!"

"Oh no, you don't!" yells Gran, leaping out of the trees behind him. "Pofs," she calls, holding up her orange like an Olympic torch, "follow me!" The wide-eyed Pofs haul up the hose and drag it back out. They charge past Brix, avoiding his glare, and hover after Gran. "To the desalination tank!"

Good idea, Gran. Why didn't Brix just do that! Why make dirty water when you could make clean, drinkable water instead?

We run off the bridge to stop Brix as he turns to escape, when Gump climbs up his body and wraps himself round the Conqip's face! Brix rattles his head and throws his arms about, trying to shake off the sloth, until finally she releases her grip and dangles off his arm. He tries dragging her back off through the trees with him, but a tiny green critter leaps out of her fur and straight into his gawking mouth. Brix screams, dropping Gump before catapulting himself into the bushes. We rush to check she's okay, then chase after Brix scrambling all the way to the Isle of Brix tunnel.

He stops at the entrance of his tunnel and dives in. We let him go. The sound of howls and heavy footsteps echo out as he legs it off down the tunnel back to his island.

14

POOP ATTACK

"We should get to the others, before Brix gets back and finds his tower flattened!"

"And the sloths," says Moojag, pressing Gump's nose like a pre-Surge door buzzer. Gump keeps on grinning, but she's frozen still. She hates that.

We fly back up to the Fort. Dad and Shenbie are standing there, surrounded by a snuggle of sleepy sloths. Aldon is missing. Travis, too.

"Brix got out," says Dad.

"We know," I say.

"He had Gump—" says Moojag.

"A critter in her fur freaked him out, though," I add, "and he took off without her back to the Isle of Brix!"

Dad sighs. "Oh dear. Gran went chasing after him!"

"She's okay," I say. "We saw her down by the river, stopping him from dumping waste water into it!"

Dad places a hand on his chest and shakes his head. "What next!"

"The tower's down," exclaims Moojag, with a somersault.

Shenbie steps forward. "Well," he says, "that's good news, at least." He peers down at Gump. "But this one's looking more frazzled than the last time I had the pleasure?"

"You would too," says Moojag, "if you got thrown about by a blockhead."

Gump slinks across the ground to the other sloths and curls herself around a tiny, meeping one. It sounds like a baby goat.

"Or if you'd lost a cute, grinning baby," I add. I've never lost a baby, but we did lose Moojag, and I know that made Dad really sad. Mum, too. Some animals don't seem to care all that much about their kids. Megapodes leave chicks to fend for themselves. Lizards forget where they've even left their eggs. Knowing me, I'd probably lose mine, too. Moojag definitely would. Some people don't even have any of their own eggs to lose. And kooky cuckoos give their eggs to other birds to hatch! I guess some people just weren't born to be parents. Some just don't want to be one, and that's cool, too. Maybe that's why the cuckoos share theirs?

"Talking of blockheads," says Shenbie, "Aldon marched Travis off to the dock to get him to unwittingly release the neurodivergents."

"And somehow," adds Dad, "he persuaded him to free all the captured sloths, too!"

Moojag starts counting the super-still creatures. Their little round eyes dart from side to side, following his every move as he hops between them. "All present," he announces, leaping back.

Gump's baby is lucky. Some animals reject their babies once humans have touched them. Dad says it's because they get scared off, or that the babies just smell different. But these sloths are used to people. Well, Conqips and Pofs, anyway.

"We have to stop him," I say, "before he does any more damage." Shenbie glares back at me. "Brix, I mean."

"Better head for the pipe, then," says Dad.

Shenbie salutes him. "Right, well, I'd best go fetch Nem Avti, before she gets lost."

"*Au revoir,* Shenbie," says Moojag, zooming off with two sloths tucked under each arm.

Is he taking them back to the trees? "Wait for us!"

"Bring the others!" he cries back.

Dad and I bend down to hoist up the remaining six. "Careful not to drop one," I say, seeing Dad wobble as the sloths cling on to his shoulders for dear life. With Gump perched on mine, and baby sloth gripping onto the fur of her back, she weaves her clawed fingers through my hair, securing them in place like a pin. The last sloth pulls themselves up my leg, clinging to it as though it's a tree trunk!

Smothered in sloth, we swing our heavy arms and legs forward, at sloth pace, after Moojag. But he doesn't turn for the woods—he just keeps on in the same direction.

"He's headed straight for Brix's tunnel, Dad!"

"What's he up to?"

Gump tugs at my hair. Her bottom starts to wiggle, and her baby lets out a high-pitched squeak.

"*Vite, vite,*" calls Moojag. "They're ready to drop a *deuce*."

I don't even have the time to describe the look on Dad's face, with the sloths getting restless and the cheeky one attached to my leg slipping off. I lift my knees as high as they can go. It feels like I'm running in slow motion.

We finally reach the entrance to the tunnel and Moojag jumps straight in. "Throw them down!" he shouts, dropping to the bottom. But they climb off and fall in without any help from us. We dive in after them and watch as they crawl on their tummies, limbs splayed, several metres down the tunnel. "Sloth attack," says Moojag, hovering back toward us with Marcel still dangling off his arm. "To stop Brix in his evil tracks!"

The sloths lever themselves up and squat a few feet apart, equally spaced along the tunnel. The one farthest starts shaking their booty, swaying from side to side, to release a ton of poop almost as tall and wide as their own body! They drag themselves up the tunnel's curved wall, skirting around the sloth in front of them, to head back up to us at the end of the tunnel. We pinch our noses, as all the sloths repeat this process, until the tunnel is filled with a load of stinky, fishy-smelling poop hills.

Moojag ferries us, one by one, out of the well. "Brix won't come back out now," he declares, gently raising Marcel's claw for a high-five.

"Can't he still come by boat?" I ask.

"At least this buys us some time," says Dad, raising a brow at my brother's pouty face.

That is a peculiar thing to say, really, when we already have all the time in the world. Plus, it doesn't cost a thing. At least, *now* it doesn't, anyway. What was it Dad used to tell us? Pre-Surgers were 'always buying time', but however much money they had, they 'seemed to constantly be running out of it'. How did they even make money? What was it made of? Did they actually swap it, like we swap avocados?

"AHHHHH!!!" echoes a horrified Conqip cry from deep inside the tunnel. "Where the devil has all this horrendous, stinking muck come from!.."

15

TURNING TRAVIS

With Brix out of the picture for now, we head back to the dock and find Aldon lecturing Travis outside Phil's Phish Bar.

"Travis, my dear. You've always been a loyal subject." The cowering Conqip only squints at him and bobs his head meekly. "As for Brix, well, he's a bit of a disappointment, isn't he. Unfit to rule *any* island, I'd say." Travis frowns. "You know, he tells everyone you're *useless*." Poor Travis, that must really hurt. He peers over his sagging shoulders at us and frowns at our reaction. I bite my lip and glance at Moojag.

"You're wrong!" he cries, flinging his arms in the air and turning away.

"He only cares about himself," I say. "But it

doesn't matter, anyway, because *you're* the boss now."

Travis swings back round and cocks his head. "Why? What's happened to my dear Brix?"

Dad steps forward. "Let's say he's having a bit of trouble with a number two."

Travis' jaw drops. "What? But he doesn't *do* number twos!"

"Of course he does," exclaims Moojag. "*Everybody* does. You could die if you didn't."

"Travis," whispers Aldon.

"Yes, A'?" utters Travis.

"Brix is not your friend."

"He's not? But—"

"And, as the niece said, you are in charge now."

"Oh! Right," Travis answers with a snortle. He glances at us and back at Aldon. "Well, I suppose I—"

"So you'll be wanting to release the Auts, then?" suggests Aldon.

"Will I?" Travis squints back at Aldon nodding. "And that would be because—"

"Because they can help you clean up Brix's mess?" Which mess?! Travis clasps his hands and paces in front of the bar. "They could even design you your very own island." His eyes widen.

"You could call it 'Travis World'," I add.

He jolts back and starts to draw a big invisible sketch in the air. "Oh, and... yes... and... How marvellous—"

"Let's have a chat with them, shall we," says Aldon, nudging him over to the doors.

"All right, fine," says Travis, pulling a long chain from his trouser pocket and jangling a bunch of keys in front of Phil's face. Phil points to the big, long, rusty key. Travis nods and steps forward to stick it in the keyhole.

Clunk! Click!

But there are two more padlocks to open. He sifts through the smaller keys, holding each up in the dim light to find the right one, until he finally starts to unlock them both.

Clunk! Click!

Click! Clunk!

Phil drags away the chains letting the double doors swing open and a swath of sweaty, sloth-like Auts spill out onto the boardwalk.

Adam and Izzy! "Hey," I say, kneeling down beside them. "Are you okay?"

"Don't know," mutters Izzy, "no PIE, no idea!"

"She's fine," says Adam, climbing off the floor. "What have we missed?" I raise my brows and shake my head.

"She's all right," says Moojag, looking Izzy over. "A snack, maybe?"

"Definitely," says Izzy. "Who's the man with the fruit?"

I look round to find Shenbie stood behind me, holding out an orange. "Uncle Shenbie. Long story," I say, as he hands it to her and pats her shoulder. "But he seems to remember *you*."

"How could I forget such a cute little face. And who's this lovely lady with the long black hair?" he asks, turning to Mum.

"It's Zoe," she says, holding out her hand.

He stares at her as though he's seen a ghost. I nod. "Well, I never."

"We talked to the Auts," she says, turning to me with a wink.

"That's right," says Phil. "They have some very interesting facts to share with Travis."

The Conqip perks up. "Go on..." he says, leaning

forward and cupping a hand to his ear.

A group of bright-eyed Auts dive in to educate a delighted Travis on the wonderful and curious history of his name. They weave in fictional stories of brave ancestors 'traversing' the universe. While another reels off a list of every single famous Travis there ever was (in chronological order—logically), Moojag and I head into the bar to search for the missing two-thirds of the Wrinkly Old Bones.

"Where did all the servants go, dear?" someone calls from behind the bar. "The service in here is absolutely despicable," they add, "even worse than in that sticky basement." Stella!

"It must be time for eggs 'n' cheese, no?" echoes a woman's voice.

"Sophia?" I call.

"Over here," answers a round behind, her arms and head still stuck inside the fridge.

"What's keeping my boy, Brix?" asks Stella. "We'll be embarrassingly late for tea with Prince William!"

"He's not coming," I whisper, gazing down at them over the bar.

"Nem Avti's girl? Is that you?"

"Yes. You're free now, you can leave."

"Oh, my dear, you're very kind but I can assure you, I have *always* been free. Free to do exactly as I please. You do realise who I am, now, don't you?"

I nod as Moojag helps them climb out. "Brix is held up," I explain, "but Izzy and Adam are right outside."

The grannies' faces light up. "What are we waiting for, then?" cries Stella, holding out their hand. "Take us to the children!"

"Where's Nem Avti?" Sophia asks softly, as we join the others.

"She's over there, with Mum and Dad."

"Goodness gracious me," says Sophia, nodding. "You've brought in *all* the troops today!"

"Indeed," adds Stella. "Only my precious Brix appears to be missing. He must be on some extra special mission. He's in charge, you know—"

"Actually," utters Travis, waltzing over, "that would be *moi*."

Stella laughs in his face. "Not you, surely, Quiffy?" they say. "You little bullies never did quite match up to my perfect boy." Wow, they really don't know their son.

"Your Isaac, dear," cries Gran, waving her arms in the air, "is the one behind the stolen money!"

Stella's face drops. Have they finally remembered the truth about their son? "Why is everyone calling him Brix?"

"That's what he calls himself, now," I explain.

"Yes, yes, I know that," they say, tutting and shaking their head at Gran. "So, where is he? Is he all right?"

"Don't worry about him," says Shenbie, stepping forward.

"You!"

"Stella," he says, with a nod. "You haven't changed a bit."

"Of course I haven't," they mutter, turning to Sophia. "But *he* has!"

"Didn't think we'd ever see *his* face again," whispers Sophia, peeking back at him. "Not here, and not after what he did to you and Isaac."

WAIT, WHAT? So who is this Shenbie?!

16

ADAM'S DAD

"I'm sorry, Stella," says Shenbie. "It wasn't easy saying goodbye."

I look over at my friend Adam. He's shaking his head at Stella. Wait... Is Shenbie Adam's grandad? "What is it with all the men in our family!" he says, ogling the man. "At least *yours* is all right," he says, stepping over to me and nodding at Dad.

"You made your choice," Stella tells Shenbie. "We can't *all* be heroes."

Dad places his hand firmly on Shenbie's shoulder. "Someone had to stay behind to protect London Tops—and the neurotypicals."

Bit weird calling them the neuro*typicals*, when there's less of them than the Real Worlders. Aren't *we* the neurotypicals, now? Or does it make *them* the neurodivergents?

"Why have you come?" asks Stella.

"The Conqips have been digging tunnels and fracking Box Hill for oil and gas," explains Shenbie. "They burrowed all the way to London Tops! So, you see, we're connected again."

Stella raises a brow at him and turns to Gran with a sigh. "Fine, just make sure he keeps his distance. Now, where is my son? I'm sure he's sorry and he'll clear all this up in a minute."

"*Our* son," answers Shenbie, "has been held up by a bunch of very slick sloths." Stella's eyes widen and their brows shoot up.

"He'll find his way back on the waters, to be sure," says Phil. "We must get it together—fast." He looks at the sky, licks his finger, and raises it up high in the air. He's doing that thing he does to feel the wind. Does feel a bit breezier than normal today. "I'd give it at least an hour before we see Brix's angry face back here." Not just his face, though—that would not be pretty!

"We've all the Auts, now," says Dad. "We just need the Pofs on side."

"What do we do with the Conqips?"

"I say we try talking them into living here with us peacefully."

"How?"

"We need to show them how good life is without all their junk food, oil, and waste."

"Maybe they could go stay on another island?" says Moojag.

Good idea. But it's no use just running away every time you don't get what you want.

"*She* did," says Moojag, glaring at Mum.

"He's right," she says. "I did. And look where that got me."

"We've done just fine," says Dad. "We couldn't all stay in London, you know that. It wasn't safe and there wasn't enough land."

"But you're all neurodivergent," says Shenbie, "of course life has been good."

"I wouldn't say it's been perfect. We might all be neurodivergent, but still, each of us is different."

"But you manage to live together."

"Yes, because we get each other," I say, "and we have enough time and space to do stuff."

Dad nods and smiles. “But I think we could accommodate a Conqip or two, couldn’t we?” I guess? Phil pouts at him, and looks back at Aldon and Travis.

“I suppose,” says Aldon, “I could spend the rest of my days here.”

Travis nods. “And very fine days they’ll be, sir.” He pats Aldon’s shoulder and mutters, “With *moi* in charge.”

Aldon tuts and leans over to whisper in my ear, “In charge of litter-picking, more likely.”

“What’s that?” I whisper back. I don’t think we have any of whatever *litter* is.

“Fruit-picker, then?” We can always do with more fruit-pickers. I nod.

“Travis,” calls Dad. “Can you round up the Conqips on the island, tell them you’re the boss now and that the party plans are off?”

“I see,” he says, hands on hips. “They won’t like it.”

“Just tell them Brix has ordered local food,” says Phil, “and they’re needed down at the dock for a spot of Frankenfishing.”

“Oh, good. Yes, they’ll enjoy that.”

"Right, that's the Conqips out of the way," says Dad. "Now what about the Pofs?"

"Oranges," says Shenbie. "I'll take them with me to harvest all the oranges at London Tops. Who's coming with?" He looks at Stella.

"*Hmmm*. I'm too old for that."

"Nonsense," says Gran, "just wear PIE."

"Where are the PIEs, Travis?" I ask.

"Can't possibly divulge that information."

"You won't be in charge any longer if you don't," says Aldon.

"They're stashed in an old trunk at Swiss Cottage."

"Home of fine Scot inventor," asks Gran, "Logie Baird's place?"

"Indeed," replies Aldon. "Brains behind the good old mechanical television. None of this PIE nonsense."

That's what we'll do! Get all the Conqips in e-skins. So they can see how easy and fun life is with PIE. "Let's go," I tell Moojag. He nods and picks me up to throw me over his shoulder. "Let's take back our *nonsense,*" he exclaims, as we wave goodbye.

17

BRIX RETURNS

"How many are there?" I ask, as Moojag flings all the PIE skins out of the chest. Nestled inside the narrow hallway of Swiss Cottage, the dark solid wood box, full of PIE, has circular images of cicadas carved into its front three panels.

"Three hundred and seventy-four," he says, finally, skipping around the neat piles of PIE on the floor.

"That ought to cover it."

"*Super*," he says, gathering them all up with two big sweeps of his muscly arms. He waits for me to climb on to his back then springs open his cicada wings. Back to dock we go.

By the time we reach the water side, everyone has disappeared and the bar is empty.

"Rat!" screams Moojag, dumping the PIEs on the

floor.

"It's okay, we'll find them."

"*Non,*" he whispers, pointing to the bar.

Oh! What's that moving? I take a step closer. It's not a rat. It's a scruffy tuft of hair bobbing up along the edge of the bar. "Travis?"

"*Shhh,*" hisses the Conqip, wriggling his stubby fingers either side of the spike of hair. "Down here!"

"TRAVIS!!!" yells a furious man's voice coming from outside. BRIX!

We dash behind the bar with all the PIEs and crouch beside Travis as the mean man stomps in, sloshing his big wet feet across the wooden floor. "WHERE ARE YOU AND WHERE ARE MY AUTS?!!!"

A quivering Travis crawls around us, pulls himself up, and creeps out in front of the bar.

"So sorry," he utters, clasping his hands. "Please forgive me, Brix. We were tricked. I don't know where they've gone."

"You mean *you* got tricked!" Travis' shoulders sag as he shakes his head. "I suppose *I'll* have to find them now," Brix groans. "I do have a way for you to redeem yourself, though," he adds, with a smirk.

"Yes, of course, B', *anything*."

"Get down to Brix Tunnel and start cleaning up the mess. Leave not a single stain behind, or there'll be no partying for you, old man!"

Eww. Poor Travis is on poop cleaning duty. "Okay, sir," he says, scrunching up his nose. I guess he doesn't know *whose*. "Oh dear," he mutters.

"What is it now, you nitwit?"

"It's just that they freed all the sloths, B'."

"They did WHAT?! You mean *you* lost them?"

"Not exactly," grumbles Travis. "It's Aldon. The man has a way with words, doesn't he?"

Brix grunts. "If I hear that vile, scrawny man's name again, I shall vomit… all over YOU..." He swears on like a machine gun, marching back out into the woods.

"If he doesn't find the sloths," warns Travis, shivering, "he'll blow the whole place up with his dynamite!"

"But we found the dynamite," I explain. "And Wats hid it all in a safe place."

"You had better retrieve it before Brix does," says Travis, flopping back down on the floor. "Because he surely will."

"We need Wats, then."

"I don't know," answers Moojag. "What do we need?"

"No, *Wats*—our friend who has a habit of turning up just when you need him."

"*Justement*," calls Moojag, darting out to a blue-striped yacht docked in the harbour. That's not one of our boats.

"Give peace a chance, man..." chants a dedicatedly merry Scot, popping up from behind the wheel. "Give peace a chance!"

"Wats!" I call, as Travis follows me out onto the deck. "Where did you stash the dynamite? We have to get it back before Brix finds it and blows up *this* island, too!"

"That fool on the hill?" he asks, pointing to a figure stumbling in our direction. Brix is headed back—*much* too soon. Wats dives down behind the wheel and we jump in and hide, leaving Travis quaking on the boardwalk.

"TRAVIS!!!" yells Brix from the woods. "You IMBECILE! Why is my tunnel STILL FULL OF STINKING SLOOP???!!!" *Sloop*. Good one. He knows a 'sloop' is a boat, though, right?

"Oh dear," Travis whimpers to himself, frozen on the spot. "I'm well and truly finished."

"There are no Auts in sight!" shouts Brix as he steps onto the harbour. "The Pofs have deserted us, to goodness-knows-where, and there's not even a whiff of Aldon and those disgusting divergent numbskulls."

We do *not* have numb skulls, thank you very much. And anyway, skulls can't be numb, they don't have a single nerve in them!

"Pure bone," whispers Moojag. "Numb-scalp or numb-brain, *sur*."

Wait—why's it gone quiet? "Are Brix and Travis still here?" I whisper.

Moojag peeps up over the rim of the boat. "*Non.*"

"They couldn't have just vanished."

"Well, they have," he says, turning to Wats. "Beatles-friend, tell us, sir, where did you hide the explosives?"

"There's a place!" Wats answers, simply.

"And that place *is*..?"

"Honey Pie, I've got a feeling that place is... Blue Jay Way."

"Jay Way?" asks Moojag.

"It's the sweetest spot," I say. "A tiny cove on the west side of the island with crystal clear blue waters, forever trapped under a lingering fog."

"Don't you be very long..." calls Wats, leaping out onto the dock and pointing out to sea. "Here comes the sun!"

"He's right," I tell Moojag. "Soon it'll get too dark to see anything over there." Wait. If the sun's coming, it won't be dark, will it?

"Where exactly did you put it?" my brother asks, as we climb out of the boat. The sun *is* coming, but of course it'll get dark before it gets light again. Is that what he meant?

"Look for the sparkly fossils, dear Lucy," Wats answers, scanning the place before flitting away.

18

BLUE JAY WAY

"It's just behind there," I call out, as Moojag flies us round the island's western corner toward a huge glowing rock. It's covered in the luminescent fossils Wats was chanting about. Moojag flaps his wings to set us down on a narrow strip of sandy beach but zooms straight back up again. "*Wait*—where are we going!"

"Brix," he whispers.

What! How is that Conqip here now, too? That crafty man has beaten us to it, and brought Travis with him. "They must've hidden on the dock and overheard us."

"And he's found the dynamite!" says Moojag, hovering us behind the rock and out of sight. Brix and Travis were standing beside a big bundle of stripy dynamite. The same lot Wats stayed behind on the Isle of Brix to get rid of, with the help of the Peace Gajooms!

An engine revs as a speedboat takes off past us. Brix is driving it, alone, with the big bunch of dynamite. And he's left Travis behind!

"Come on," I say, nudging my brother. He flinches. "Sorry," I say.

"All right," he answers, with a nod. But I know it's not. If he had PIE, he wouldn't have felt a thing with Sensory Seeker mode turned off.

We fly back round. "Ah!" calls Travis, waving us down. "He sent you back for me!"

"No," I call, as Moojag wobbles to land beside the frowning Conqip on a bumpy carpet of smooth black pebbles. "But we will happily give you a lift if you tell us exactly where Brix is taking that dynamite!"

Travis sticks his hands on his hips and gazes out to sea. "Take one last gander," he says with a pout and shaking his head. "It's the last time any of us will take in this splendid view."

Moojag glares at Travis as I grab the man's shoulder. "Where is he going to detonate the explosives?" My brother squints at me and then at the Conqip, too.

"Detonation Station, of course," answers Travis. Moojag and I turn to each other and burst out laughing. "What *now*," he says, tilting back his head.

"Detonation Station," I say. "Really?"

"Yes? And what is so darn funny about that?" Moojag can't control his giggles. He may never be able to stop. He might keep laughing till his head blows off. Not literally, of course. Get it together, girl. Stop! "You know, the old Visitor Centre," declares Travis, with a sigh.

"You mean," I say, choking back a giggle, "those brick buildings next to the Fort?" Travis nods. "Okay. I know a shortcut."

"Better not be a short fuse, too," Moojag says, jellyfishing my hand instead of bumping it. He grabs Travis' arm and propels us up with a spin. I point to the north-east, in the direction of Detonation Station, and we're off again, with Travis clinging on for dear life. Wait. Short fuse? Ah—the dynamite.

As we fly over the woods, there's a loud rustling from below. We look down and see a stream of Real Worlders winding out of the woods through the trees. "Hey," I call to them. "Where are you all going?"

The group at the front have sloths clung to their

backs like backpacks. “We’re taking them to the Visitor Centre,” someone yells back up.

“It’s over there,” calls Travis, pointing to the red buildings near the Old Fort. But as we get closer, he yells “Nooooo! Turn back!”

Brix is down there, standing at the building’s front entrance, the bundle of Gajoomstik dynamite by his feet.

“Land us on the roof,” I say, as Moojag swerves round the back of the building. He hovers up onto the roof and plants us at its outer edge so we can peer down at Brix without him spotting us. “What’s he got in his hand?” I whisper.

Moojag’s eyes widen. “*Mèches*,” he whispers loudly. I frown as he glares back at me. “MATCHES—thin wooden sticks with tips that catch fire when you rub it against a rough surface. ‘Safety’ matches need a special surface to light. ‘Strike-anywhere’ matches—well, you can figure that out for yourself, sis.”

“I know what a match is, bro.” And Brix is ready to light the dynamite with one. “We don’t want to be here if that dyno’s about to blow!”

“Why would he light it?” says Moojag. “He’d only blow himself up, too.” True.

"Excuse me," says Travis, squeezing his head between us, "but Master Brix does have the helicopter." He points to the roof of the building next door. There really is a helicopter. So he thinks he can run all the way up there and fly away before that stuff detonates?

"He runs pretty fast, actually," says Moojag. "When he wants." L-A-Z-Y Conqips. Always in a hurry.

Makes sense. Dad used to say pre-Surgers were 'always in a rush, so they never got the chance to appreciate anything'. Especially the neurotypicals. Because they 'never made space to really think about what they were doing, or enjoy what they had'. Most of them only cared 'how they looked, and ignored what they actually felt inside'. Is Brix really thinking about what he's doing right now? Or is his plan literally going to blow up in his own pretty face?

"Here they come!" exclaims Moojag, as a bunch of sloth-carrying, Brix t-shirt-wearing Real Worlders army-crawl like sloths round the back of the building. They stop at the corner and let our new mossy friends slip off and roll all the way round to Brix's feet—and the dynamite!

19

DYNAMITE FART

The sloth at the front of the sloth gang drags their body forward to park themselves right beside Brix. The cringing Conqip glares down at them, then turns to pull a single matchstick from the box. I wince as he lifts his foot to strike it against the heel of his shiny black shoe. They'd better not be 'strike-anywhere' matches! I glance at Moojag already nodding back at me.

Cupping his hand around the flame, Brix carefully lowers the match. I shake my head and glance away, but Moojag pokes me, so I look back. The sloth has swung round and stuck their bum in the air, right up in front of Brix. The flame is ready to lick the wick, when... *Pffft!* and then—

POW! — a sloth fart explosion

catapults Brix right up onto our roof!

He has somehow crash-landed on all fours next to us without a single scratch. I grip the rooftop's outer ledge and lean over to check on the sloths down below. They look a bit frazzled, but they're also fine. The Real Worlders are gathering around them. Some are carrying the neurodivergents who can't walk now, not without their PIE skins to support them: the ones who arrived on Box Hill in a wheelchair but walked ever since they got their hands on one of Gran's PIEs. Others are struggling to move in their tight, figure-hugging Brix t-shirts. They haven't needed clothes made for them since the day they proudly donned the size-inclusive skins.

I turn back to Brix, who's pulling away from Travis patting his shoulder like he's his pre-Surge pet dog.

Wait! Since when do sloths fart? "I thought they couldn't do that?" Brix nods, frowning hard.

"Me three," adds my brother.

"Indeed they can," answers Travis.

Brix glares back at him. "You didn't know that."

"I did, actually!" he says, grinning and looking very pleased with himself. "Zoologists assumed they couldn't until the summer of 2025 in Costa Rica, when

Bräutigam witnessed one trumping away in the bath."

"Well," says Brix, massaging his hip. "A little poop and fart isn't going to stop *me*." A little?

"What ya gonna do?" says Moojag, arms crossed.

"Out of my way, Buzby," he says, poking my brother and pushing past us all. "This ain't over."

Brix gazes down at all the Real Worlders, then over at the building next door—and the helicopter! He glances back at us with his slimy grin, then turns to make a run for it. He's not actually going to jump, is he? We all stare, open-mouthed, as he takes a giant leap off the roof! He just makes it onto the other building, landing *splat!* face down, with his legs still hanging off the edge. *Ouch.*

"I'm okay!" he calls back, craning his neck and dragging himself up.

"*Bah*," mutters Moojag. Right. Like we care if the guy who's gonna destroy us is fine. Moojag glances at me and crosses his arms. But Brix is Adam's dad. Wait—maybe Adam can stop him, once and for all?

The Real Worlders are shouting up at us now. I look down at them all. Dad's there with them, throwing his arms about. Adam and Izzy, too.

"He's got a helicopter!" I call down. "On the other

building—"

"We're on our way!" Dad calls back.

"Brix," I call over, "where are you going?"

"Like he's gonna tell!" says Moojag. What's with all the 'gonnas' today? He chuckles and whispers, "He's not *gonna* get very far without his dynamite, or the tower."

Brix taps his nose and yells, "Never you mind, Real Nerders." He turns to climb into the helicopter just as Dad steps out onto the roof, panting, having raced up the stairs.

What if Brix has more explosives somewhere else?! Moojag and I rush down, into the other building, and run up the stairs to the roof.

"Hold it!" says Dad, bent over with his hands on his knees, as we join the others.

"What for?" answers the gloating Conqip. "The world is my oyster now!" Well, that's just silly. How is the world an oyster?

Moojag shakes his head. "And why would it be *his*, even if it ever did turn into one!" I love that my brother can hear everything I'm thinking, but sometimes it might be nice to just keep my thoughts to myself. Especially the weird ones. You know?

"And what about your son?" says Dad, pointing to Adam.

"Dad," says Adam, walking towards his father.

"What's he doing here!" groans Brix.

"You don't have to do this," says Adam, as we step over together. "Everybody loves you." Stretching it a bit, my friend.

"Love," says Brix, pouting, "what's that?"

"Your mum loves you," I call out. "So you must know what love is."

He throws his head back with a cackle. "That stuck-up lady only ever cared how much money anyone had."

"Like you, you mean?" I ask. Brix ponders for a moment and cackles some more.

"I'm no 'lady'," bellows Stella, striding out the doorway and across the roof. They step up to Brix and hold out their hand. "As I have already informed you, son, it's they/them."

"Whatever," he says, crossing his arms.

"Just as you are now called 'Brix', and not 'Isaac' anymore."

"Well," he says. "*You* don't care, so—"

"Of course they do," says Dad. "As does Shenbie."

"Shen-*who*?"

"Grandad," explains Adam.

Brix looks round in terror at Shenbie. At *his* dad! The whole lot of them are up here now, trying to stop him.

Surrounded, Brix backs up into the helicopter's cockpit and slams the door shut in Shenbie's face. He glances back through the window at Adam with barely a nod, and starts the engine. We run from the launchpad as the helicopter's blades start to spin and it hovers up. A nod is a good sign, though. Isn't it? He must love his son, surely? He's not a cuckoo.

"What's that—" shouts Dad, as we all cover our ears, "hanging off the landing skid?"

20

SAVING BRIX, SAVING BOX HILL

A brave sloth has climbed onto one of the helicopter's landing skids and is dangling off the left arm. These creatures can hang for hours and hours with their super strong upper limbs!

Brix tries taking off in the direction of the dismantled tower, but the helicopter tips with the sloth swinging back and forth. Trying to get up into the cockpit, they plaster themselves over the windscreen instead. Brix sticks his head out of the window to yell, "Get off my copter, slimeball..!" But the sloth won't let go. "And wipe that stupid grin off your face!" The helicopter starts to turn, spinning all the way round before plummeting down the back side of the building.

"He's lost control!" calls Dad, turning to us. Yep. Nothing new there.

"Come on," shouts Shenbie.

"We're coming, too," I say, seeing Adam turn back and cross his arms.

"I'll go. For the sloth," he says, peering at me, over his shoulder. I nod.

We bolt down the stairs after Dad and Shenbie and run out the open doorway. The helicopter is hovering there, just above the ground.

"Show's over," yells Shenbie, waving Brix down.

The Conqip shakes his head violently. "*Arrrgggh,*" he growls. "Why can't you weirdos just leave me alone!"

"Because," calls Stella, "like it or not, you're a weirdo, too!"

I nod. *Weirdo*, *weirdo*, *weirdo*. Adam just tuts. Izzy jumps in to stare up at Brix. "You do look a bit alike," she says, turning to Adam with a grin. "More hair though," she adds, poking his shoulder.

"Not now, Izzy," he says, nudging her away.

"Well," she continues, "he *is* your Dad."

"Unfortunately."

"Don't be like that," I say. "Sometimes good

people do bad things."

"Sometimes?" Adam whispers, hands on hips. "I'm ashamed to be that meanie's son."

"Go on," I say, prodding him. "Talk to the man. He's not *all* mean. And he's a fast runner!" Maybe he doesn't remember that though?

"*All right*—if that's what it takes to stop all your nagging." He steps cautiously up to the floored helicopter, while Izzy and I stride over to the sloth and coax them away with the carob leaves I saved for Marcel and Gump. They slide off the windscreen and land on their back.

"Here you go," says Izzy with a smile. "I bet these are your favourite! I love carobs. They're so sweet. Especially when they're fresh. All oozy and juicy like honey!" The creature flips over onto their front and taps the floor. I drop a leaf. They stab it with their claw, raise it to their mouth, and take a lick. That could be all they can digest in one go. Izzy drops another leaf and steps back after me. The sloth eyes the leaf then turns their head right round. Checking for their sloth family?

"They're on the other side," says Izzy. I frown at her. She smiles. "Yes, I know—they don't speak English."

"They don't speak, *point final*—full stop," says

Moojag.

"Well, they don't need to," I add.

"Do *you*?" replies Moojag.

True. But not everyone is psychic like us.

"Goodbye!" shouts Brix. Wait, what?! The man is being swept away by a couple of Conqips!

"Where'd *they* come from?" asks Izzy.

"They just appeared out of nowhere!" Somewhere, Adam. *Somewhere.*

"Collect the dynamite," cries Stella, grabbing a bunch of PIEs. "And hand out the rest of these!" They swing round to Shenbie. "Time to find my friend, Nem Avti, and get these PIEs on the Conqips, pronto!"

We wave goodbye to Stella and Shenbie, then start sifting through PIEs to get everyone back into their skin.

"Not mine," mutters Sparkles, shaking her head. She turns to her brother, Sparky. He frowns, points to himself and flicks his hand out from under his chin. "Not *his*, either!"

This is impossible. Auts, like sloths, need extra time and space to process things. But this lot have had a taste of their very own PIEs, so they probably feel like they can't live without them! I know slow isn't lazy, Gran, and, yes, it's a survival strategy—but right now we don't have much time at all! Moojag nods. And, hopefully, this is only temporary. "I'm really sorry, Auts," I say, "but it's going to have to be a different PIE—"

"Or *no* PIE." calls Moojag. Harsh.

Sparky's eyes widen, as his sister snatches up two random PIEs.

"It's just for one day," I reassure them all. Moojag clasps his hands. "You'll get your own PIEs back once the Conqips are converted!" The Auts chatter amongst themselves for a minute, then nod back. Each collects a PIE and pulls the skin up over their Brix shirt. Some cover their heads, too, sighing as their shoulders drop with the hoods massaging their tensed-up necks. Recharged and armed with a fresh load of 'spoons', everybody raises a fist in the air, and, like a swarm of determined bees, we all chase off together after Stella and Shenbie.

Sparky sprints ahead at sonic speed. "Not a race," calls Moojag, zooming up on the inside to lead the way.

"But it's so much fun!" cries Sparkles. Sparky flaps his arms and spins round with a smile. "I've never seen him like this before," she calls, skipping along. "What are we going to do to the Conqips?" she asks with a pout, as we catch up.

"We're going to give them a taste of PIE," I answer. "Chill them out."

Sparkles grins. "Well," she says, stroking my twinkling gold arm, "They aren't that yummy, but they do *feeeel* amazing." I nod.

Everyone looks so happy, the Real Worlders and the Auts, too. Some have smiles on their faces; others glow so bright on the inside, you can just feel it. But it's too much, so I raise my hood and nod to Moojag. I call, "*Sensory Seeker off*," at Spondylux, and wait for my hood to fully inflate. And just like that, everything is right. The sounds, smells, feels. It's all still there, just softer, with only a single voice in my ear at a time.

Moojag swerves, hovering to Dad's side. "Jack…"

Our father stops and waits for my brother to find the words.

"Can we really?"

"What's that, Moojag?"

"Live with them, *justement*?"

"We can try. Can't we?"

Moojag scrunches up his face and glances at me.

I hunch my shoulders and gaze back at all the pale,

freshly-freed Auts pottering on. Maybe the Conqip can. But can *they*?

21

BACK TO SWISS COTTAGE

"Girl!" calls Gran, speeding toward us, with a bunch of Peace Gajooms in tow. "This way!" I press my skin to turn Sensory Seeker back on and wave.

"We're coming, Nem Avti," I call, as Dad waves on the others and takes my hand.

"These Mights will round up the sloths," says Gran, reaching us.

"Ask me why!" shouts Wats, leaping out in front of her from somewhere.

"Wats!" I call back.

"Not *what*, why!" Oh dear, not him now, too.

"Okay," I say, with a sigh, "why?"

"Because," he answers, "I know you know my name!"

Wait, what? "No. You asked us *why*."

"Just act naturally," he says, pacing about. Moojag hovers behind me. "Brix has been a bad boy. Not bad to me, per se…" Probably not English, but sounds good—so who cares. "Your mother should know," he says, leaping in front of Dad. "But she forgot to remember to forget!" Oh my goodness me. Should someone help him out?

"Did you want to ask something?" Dad says softly.

Wats pauses for a moment, pressing a finger to his lips. "Ask me why!" he says, scissor-kicking his legs and swinging both arms out to the side.

"Why?"

"*Because*—only the Goo Goo G'jooms can carry all that weight!" That's it? I chuckle to myself and shake my head.

Gran eyes up Dad and steps over to Moojag. "Who is this man, Jack?"

"I am Moojag," he answers. "*He* is your son, Jack."

"Are you sure?" she says, peering into Dad's face. "How old does that make me, then?"

I smile at her and say, "As old as you feel, Nem Avti?"

"That's right!" she exclaims, wide-eyed. "29!

Sweet girl, how did you know?"

"Mum told us. But what happened to Uncle Aldon? And Travis?"

"They're quite safe, don't you worry your little head about them. We're having a little trouble with Brix, though. That's Stella's boy, Isaac. But he's Brix now."

"Yes," I say. "We know."

"Ye know too much!" Well, yes, maybe. "Let's go, troops," she says. "Onward, and quite *literally* upwards, to Swiss Cottage!"

We all sprint after Gran in her glowing copper-gold PIE and march up the hill together to the house. Stooped under its little wood-and-tile veranda, two Conqips in black-tie guard the door.

"We're here for Isaac." The men glance at each other, cocking their heads. They look back at her and laugh.

"Brix," explains Dad.

The Conqip on the left nods, while the other shakes his head. "Nope. You're still not coming in."

"We've strict instructions," says the first, stamping his foot. "No one is to disturb his Highness." Wow. Is that what he's calling himself now!

"His Highness will *not* want to miss this," says

Gran.

They look at each other; one whispers something to the other before turning back to her. “Tell us whatever it is,” he says, almost dropping the half-filled champagne flute in his hand, “and we’ll pass on the message.”

Gran picks two of the PIEs and hands them over. “These are for you. You can keep them.”

“We don’t wear dirty nerdivergent tech.”

How very cruel. But maybe he’s a bit tipsy, and he didn’t mean to say it in a mean way? PIEs aren’t dirty, though. That’s technically physically impossible.

“I assure you,” replies Gran, “you won’t get cleaner than a PIE.”

Dad and I nod. Moojag tips his hat and holds it flat against his chest.

“This one’s idea, was it?” says the Conqip on the left, sporting a wonky bow tie. “Old Buzby?”

“Moojag!” exclaims my brother, hovering behind me.

“Hmm,” says Wonky. “I don’t think we should—”

“It has a bunch of functions,” says Dad. “If you’re feeling ill, it will check your vitamin and mineral levels, and then tell you exactly what your body needs.”

"We're not ill," says the other one. He really does look very pasty, though. Both of them do.

"You seem a bit hot, too," says Gran. "This will cool you down or stop you feeling queasy right away."

He wipes his forehead and nods to Wonky. They look the PIEs over, stroking the scaly skin. They stare for a moment, mesmerised by the hexagonal cells all lighting up, before snapping out of their daze and chucking the PIEs straight back in Gran's face. "What sorcery is this, woman!" cries Wonky.

"It's just simple coding, my dears," says Gran. "No harm came, or will come, to any being in the making of PIE."

"You activated the climate sensor," explains Dad. "Simply by thinking about it. If you put it on, you'll *feel* it, too."

Pasty holds out his hand to Gran, and points to the large-spotted green PIE. She holds it up and he nods. She hands it over and points to his shoes. "Those'll have to come off," she says, nodding as he kicks off the muddy brogues. "And the rest of your pomp," she adds, circling her wand-like finger at his dinner jacket. Cowering behind his friend, he removes his jacket and trousers. "The shorts and shirt can stay," she adds, leaning forward to help him pull the PIE up over his clothes and lift up the hood. She gives him a thumbs up as he steps out in front of the veranda. He strokes his arm, then looks back at his friend.

"You all right?" whispers Wonky.

Pasty holds a finger up and looks away for a second, then smiles. "I can't feel a thing!"

"What have you done?!" says the other one, glaring at Dad.

But it wasn't what Pasty meant. Moojag flies between them. "It is good, *oui*?"

"*Oui*," agrees Pasty, as a flock of birds soars over us—higher than I've ever seen them go before. "It's pure bliss!"

Wonky turns to his friend, placing a firm hand on his shoulder. "*Shhh.*"

Pasty gasps, then swings round to peek through the slit window. Brix must've heard us.

22

CONQIP PIE

"What's all the racket?" shouts Brix, stomping for the door.

"One moment, sir!" calls Wonky, leaning against it as Pasty attempts to strip off the PIE with one hand and collect up the strewn clothing from the floor with the other. But Brix forces it open and barges out, squashing poor Wonky between the door and the wall.

"What *are* you doing?" he yells at Pasty, who's covered up his PIE legs with the jacket. "Are you wearing nerd tech?!"

Brix unbuttons his shirt collar and wipes the sweat from his forehead. Wonky hobbles out from behind the door and sways over to him. "Apparently, it's a healing suit!"

Brix yawns, shaking his head. How has he not even

noticed any of us yet?

"That's what the Real Nerders are saying," adds Pasty, turning to us.

Brix swings round and bolts right back. "*Arrgggh.* Please tell me I'm dreaming!"

"Sorry, sir," answers Wonky.

"Nimbeciles! Why must I do *everything* around here? What good is it having guards if they can't hack the job?" Pasty clasps his hands. "No," says Brix, cocking his head and brushing the quivering Conqip away. "You're sacked!" He turns to Wonky and whispers, "Bring me a TOUGHER Conqip! We need backup. NOW."

"I'm sorry—"

"You're sorry, too? *Ugghh*—all I ever hear is SORRY. What the devil is it, man?"

Wonky points to a string of PIE-wearing men skipping toward us! Conqips? It's hard to tell out of their dinner suits. Despite the wide grins, those faces look tired, and they have sagging skin under the eyes. Most definitely *not* Real Worlders. Conqips.

Gran leaps over to Brix and presents him with a PIE.

"I don't care how many Conqips you've

brainwashed, Wrinkly Bones," he says, crossing his arms. "I shan't ever be seen in one of those!"

"Just try it on," I utter, leaning forward.

"You don't know where those things come from, do you, girl," he says, staring down at me like I very well should.

I certainly haven't been told the whole story! "Gran designed them, with Zoe and Jack," I say, looking to Dad, "for the Real Worlders." I glance back at them all gathered a few safe metres behind us, along with all the Auts.

"But did they tell you about the ZIZANTH?" he asks, shaking his head at Gran. "Naughty, naughty, Granny." Am I finally going to find out what she had to do with the nasty experiment?

I turn to Gran. "What *did* you do, Nem Avti?" I ask, dropping my head.

"It's not what you think," says Dad, stepping beside her.

She sighs, rocking her head. "I didn't know what Aldon was up to," she says. "I just gave him the money to set it up."

"Set up *what*?" I ask, shaking my head. "How could you pay for experiments on children!"

"She thought he was researching a cure for physical disabilities," says Dad.

"Okay, but what about the Auts!"

Brix laughs, patting Gran's shoulder. "There's no way Nem Avti didn't know about the nerdy Auts."

Gran shakes her head and crosses her heart. "In return for the money, Aldon gave me exclusive private access to a lab. That's where I developed PIE with my Jack and Zoe. But I didn't—"

I glare up at Dad. "You knew?!"

Dad sighs. "How were we to know Aldon was collecting Auts to rid them of their special interests and force them to hyperfocus on his project? We thought he was helping Monzi," he explains, glancing back at Moojag. "When our boy got really sick, we thought we were going to lose him. Aldon was our only hope—all the hospitals were flooded and doctors scarce."

"Oh, they *knew*," says Brix. "How could they not have noticed the nerdy Auts in there, developing our secret underground kingdom!"

"I only had access to my lab," insists Gran. "Do you really think I would've let him do that to Monzi? Our boy?" Moojag slumps down cross-legged and slams his top hat on the ground.

Of course Gran didn't know. She loves Moojag. She was probably so focused on making PIE, that if there had been a sign Aldon was up to no good, she could easily have missed it. It's no excuse. But it's a perfectly good reason.

My PIE cells start to vibrate. I've turned orange! It's okay. Just breathe. Everything will be fine. My shoulders relax as I sit down beside my brother. He nods. I hold a thumb up and he cocks his head. "Do you want a PIE?" He shakes his head and rubs the sleeve of his tailcoat jacket. Happy in his own clothes—even if they do make him itch. He swipes the sweat from his forehead. Even when he's hot, too. Wait, it does feel *really* hot right now, though. This isn't me just feeling anxious, or Moojag feeling uncomfortable. All our PIEs have started flashing red. Something's very wrong!

"Help!" calls Wats, running in our direction as a herd of deer gallops past. "Emergency on planet earth!"

Moojag whispers, "Not a Beatles song!" as I leap up.

"Revolution!" adds Wats, jumping up and down. Moojag nods. "I, Me, and Mine has started a fire!" He points to Brix and up at the bright red sun in the sky. All around us, the ground has turned a hazy orange. I cough and rub my eyes from the smoke starting to fill the air. Wats spins round and points to the woods.

The trees are on fire!

Moojag and I gasp. The sloths!

As a tear falls into my brother's lap, he dons his hat and leaps up. I tug his coattails, but he pulls them back and hovers away, flying straight for the glowing orange blaze! We cry after him, but he's already flown a third of the way to the woods. If we go, too, we could get burnt. If we don't, the sloths could die, and Moojag along with them! Has PIE ever had to protect us from anything like this before?

Everyone is just standing frozen still. I run toward Gran, but I don't feel my legs. Are they even moving?

When I finally reach her, she doesn't see me. I wave my arms in front of her face. "Nem Avti!" I cry. "HELP! What do we do?"

"Such a beautiful sunset tonight," she says, grinning. I shake my head and look round for Dad. I feel sick to my stomach. The smoke is filling the air, and our lungs, but Gran isn't seeing what's right in front of her eyes!

23

HELP!

Gran stares into the blood-red sky. She doesn't even blink.

"What's wrong with her, Dad!"

"She's scared. She doesn't want to believe what's happening, so she's escaped into her own world."

"No, Gran!" I yell at her. "It's fire! Box Hill is on fire!"

"I'll be back," calls Dad, stripping off his PIE and running back to Brix with it flying like a flag. The Conqip is half-grinning, half-terrified, surrounded by a panicked angry mob of Real Worlders. Does he realise what an awful thing he's done? Dad shoves the PIE into the man's middle. "Put this on, NOW!" he shouts at him.

"Ha!"

"It'll save you if you can't escape in time."

The ground rattles from Brix's helicopter exploding as a massive fireball erupts. Then the truck by the dismantled tower screeches. Its drum peels back like a banana and spirals up into the sky before shards of twisted metal fall, clattering onto the floor. My nostrils fill with the smell of burning oil; my ears, with a high-pitched ringing. Brix finally accepts the PIE. He gestures for the Auts to look away.

Dad sprints back and Mum hands him a new PIE. "Dishabiliophobia," he whispers in my ear.

"Let's go!" calls Mum.

"What's dipiphobia?" I ask Spondylux, running behind Dad and Mum chasing after Moojag.

DID YOU MEAN 'DEIPNOPHOBIA' — THIS IS THE FEAR OF DINING OR DINNER CONVERSATIONS.

What? That's not right. PIE must be saving energy for more important features—like saving our lives! But Brix is definitely *not* afraid of dining, or of talking to people—especially when it's a careless waste of words. Which is most of the time, to be fair.

Dad calls '*Superspeed*' and '*BurnBloc*' into

Spondylux. Burn block?

"Fear of being judged or exposed," he shouts back. What? 'Burn bloc'? That doesn't sound right. Oh, he means the *dishabi*-wotsit!

"That's why he's so *mean*," I yell, as Dad races on ahead of us, "because he's scared?" *Mean, mean, meanie.*

"Probably, my love," says Mum, synching up my PIE with hers as we keep on running. It feels as though we're going nowhere fast. Just like those pre-Surgers.

The orange glow around us is only getting brighter, with the fire chomping its way through the forest. The unrelenting flames swirl and whoosh with every slight turn of the wind. Smoke billowing up out of the tree tops. The fire is so furious now, it couldn't care less about all the tiny creatures trapped inside those woods.

Cool air flushes up my PIE and a thermal wave rises up through the hood to shield my bare face. The blazing heat must be unbearable out there. I could turn off the sound of the fire roaring, but I need to hear Mum. "It's okay, my love," she calls, grabbing my hand. "We'll rest our ears once this is all over."

I don't know what 'all over' looks like. The worst thing that's ever happened to us was the Great Surge.

That was bad. And it was years ago. An island blew up, of course, but now there's a great wall of fire right in front of us! And the thing is growing so tall and fast, and moving in so many different directions, that you can't even tell which way it's headed next.

Wait! What's that flying out of the smoke?

Moojag!

He zooms toward us with four sloths clung to his wings. I wave him down as he hovers above us. But he stalls, motioning to the trees. "Up there!" he calls. The rest of the sloths have made it all the way to the top of the highest canopy. Still grinning, but most definitely terrified. Just like Brix.

"Do you think you could wear PIE?" Dad calls, beckoning him down.

"I can do it!" Moojag answers, shaking the black powder off of his hat before handing it to me.

"Good lad," calls Dad, tears rolling down his cheeks. Complicated tears. "Take me up there!"

Mum strips off her PIE. I shake my head, but she just smiles back at me and helps my brother climb quickly into it. No time to give her mine—I scoop her up and run at the highest speed PIE can carry us.

"Get to water, Nem." I nod, but the air is thick with smoke, now. And which *way* is the sea?!

Boom! Boom!

That's not me shaking the ground!

Gajoom…stik!

Or making that sound!

Gajoom…stik!

Gajoom…stik!

"What is it?" cries Mum. She coughs, choking, as I squint through the fog for signs of Gajoom. "I've heard that before."

A vision of white and purple stripes appears through the haze. The Gajoomdom Gajooms! I leap us out of the way as the sticky robots bolt past us, heaving an endless hose. Their stripes have gone all wonky. Light purple splotches bleed out from blurred, zig-zagging lines. "It's Moojag's robots, Mum. They're going to put out the fire!"

They're all sugar, though, aren't they? What if they melt before they can even put it out!

"Not *only* sugar," calls Moojag, whizzing past us in a glittering black PIE with all the sloths hanging off one arm and Dad tucked under the other. "Only sticky on the outside." We race after him through the clearing fog, past a scurry of grey squirrels leaping over a queue of snails. Not stopping, not thinking, till we reach the harbour!

24

CONQIP LOVE

Everyone is gathered on the harbour, safe and (barely a) sound. Brix is leaning against the railing on the pier, surrounded by a group of dithering Auts. He doesn't look angry anymore, though. More sad, like a deflated balloon.

"We're not out of the woods yet," says Aldon.

We're not? I glance at the ground around my feet. Moojag shakes his head at him.

"Not literally, nephew." Oh! Moojag and I sigh. Uncle points to glowing rows of charred, hollowed-out tree trunks and black fallen branches. "The embers could get carried by the wind and spark up new fires…"

"Is everyone accounted for?" Dad calls to Gran and Phil, who are still busy counting heads.

"All here!" she answers back, tapping the last one. "And the Auts?"

"All here!" he calls back. "Right," he says. "Everyone on Myrta. We can't stay here, in any case. It's too dangerous breathing in the smoke, even with PIE."

And the Gajooms? "They will live," answers Moojag.

I run back to Gran. "The Peace Gajooms?"

"Making peace, of course," she says with a grin. What does *that* mean? "They're with Wats, spreading love to Conqips."

"So, they don't fight, then?"

"Absolutely not! Who do you think I am?"

Gran, of course.

"How do they make peace, then?"

Izzy jumps out from the crowd and hugs me. She *meant* for it to be a light one. "They spread the *loooooove*," she says, turning to her wise, wrinkly-faced gran. Sophia nods and for a moment her warm smile melts all our troubles away. She points to a circle of Conqips on the deck, locked inside a vibrating ring of jolly Peace Gajooms.

"Where's Adam?" I ask, looking round.

"With his Daddy," mumbles Izzy, munching on a

dog-nut.

"Where did you get that?"

"A Pof, of course!" says Izzy, skipping up to a small girl pushing her way through the crowd. The Pof's wings spring back up as she pops out between a couple of curious Real Worlders. It's Kitty.

"Yum yum!" says the Pof, licking her fingers.

"What have you got there?" I ask, crouching down.

"Avocado!" she exclaims, opening the palm of her other hand to reveal the stone. She lifts her arm to throw it.

"Wait," I say, "what are you doing?"

"It's trash," she answers. Like pre-Surge rubbish?

"Don't get rid of it," I say, shaking my head. "You can make all sorts of cool things from the seed!"

Kitty's eyes widen as she hovers by my side. "Snacks?"

I nod. "Delicious smoothies, avocado tea... Bread, even. And you can grow a whole new tree from the seed. Sometimes, I like a soak in an avocado bath, when I get bored of self-cleaning with PIE, of course."

"Me not wash with pie!" she says, giggling at me and shaking her head. "Me eat it!"

"Me too!" adds another Pof, hovering toward us.

She hoists up a sagging tutu full of oranges.

"Where did you get all those?" I ask.

"Shenbie Darling!" she says, flapping her wings. "From London Stops!" Fast work, Stelbie.

Gran nods. "Tops, dear," she says with a wink. "Stella has decided to move back there with Shenbie." *Really* fast work. "They'll try to convince Brix to go with them."

Probably for the best. But this, I need to see! I run over to them. I hope they won't make Adam go, too.

"Thank you," Brix tells Dad. He actually *means* it!

"Of course." Of course *what*. That we saved the man who tried to kill us all? That we gave him our own clothes, even though he destroyed everything we worked for years to build? Dad places his hand on my shoulder. "Everyone deserves a second chance, Nem." I know, but it feels like he's had more than two.

Stella and Shenbie thank the Auts for watching over their son, before the teens spread out into smaller groups and slowly make their way to Phil's Bar. They join the crowd of Real Worlders standing under the string of twinkling solar lights, as the fire in the forest dies down.

The smell of smoke and gas hits my nose again with the thermal shield dissolving away. I suck my tongue and swallow the bitter metallic taste in my mouth.

"You don't need oil," says Shenbie, "when you have solar-powered PIEs, 3D printers, and never-ending tons of pre-Surge waste to create anything new you could ever want."

Stella takes Brix's hand and places it on Shenbie's outstretched palm. "Your dad didn't stay behind because he doesn't love us, son," they explain. "He just wanted to keep the Londoners safe. He has always loved London so."

Shenbie nods, twirling his moustache. "Come with us. And you can start afresh."

Brix grimaces at his Dad's London Underground shorts and shakes his head.

"It's all over, your Highness," says Gran, skipping over. "Your plan has failed. The animals are gone, the champagne has run out, and your fellow Conqips are choosing the Real World." She points to the giddy men dancing in PIEs all colours of the rainbow. "The Pofs are done with you, too."

Brix scans the blackened island. "I only meant to scare the sloths," he whispers, gazing into the distance. "I was going to put it out."

"Come with us to London Tops," says Stella.

"Why would you want that," he says, peeking at them from the corner of his eye, "after everything I've done?"

"We love you, Brix," says Stella.

"And we have a lot of catching up to do, son," adds Shenbie.

Adam steps over to his father's side, Gump's baby clung to him like a tiny backpack. "Why did you take this poor creature from their mum?"

"I wasn't going to eat it," he says, peering at the grinning, wide-eyed creature and wiggling his finger in their face. "I only wanted to play." Brix isn't mean, he's just bored and lonely!

"You took me from mine, too, didn't you," says Adam.

"Your mother was sick. And I couldn't look after you either." Adam looks round at Stella and Shenbie nodding back. "I always had so much work, and very little time."

"But you have plenty of it, now," says Stella.

"And I'm in charge..." says Travis, sliding in

between them, "so please do take a long, well-deserved break!"

Brix raises his brow at Travis smirking, and turns to Adam. "Will you come?"

"I'll stay with my friends, thanks," says Adam. "But we'll visit," he adds, glancing back at us. I nod. Izzy and Sophia do too. Brix gazes down at the ground, shoulders slumped, then follows on after his parents, dragging his feet all the way to the harbour.

"Not a sight I thought I'd ever see," says Aldon, pouting.

Travis nods, hands on hips. "Indeed."

"You're not in charge, by the way," says Gran, waving as Stelbix sail off. "…Yes, Travis, I'm talking to *you*."

The Conqip swings round to Aldon. "But *he* said, and *she* said—"

"You've done very well, and we are grateful," she continues, nodding, "but there's never anyone in charge here." Aldon shakes his head with a sigh.

Moojag spins round, clasping his hands. "The Pofs will keep you both busy," he says, skipping off to all the winged Mights hovering excitedly around the returned

Gajooms.

"Oh, goodie," mutters Travis, rubbing his hands.

"They'll have jobs for you," I explain. "And I'm sure the Auts can find you something to do, too."

Travis squints at Aldon, then sighs. "Fine."

25

ALL YOU NEED IS PIE

"All you need is PIE!" calls Wats, setting sail on his Mystery Boat, to only Wats-knows-where, for only Wats-knows-how-long. I wave goodbye and wander back up the winding path to the viewing point. Moojag and Marcel are sitting on the wall, watching the sunrise.

"Can I?" I ask, flopping down beside them. Moojag nods and Marcel just grins, but he's not frozen still, so I think I'm okay to stay.

As I turn to look up at the sky, a black-backed woodpecker swoops down and perches on my knee. I hold still, but 'Ebony' flaps her wings and flies back to the charred woods, scavenging for more beetle juice. Half of Box Hill's trees were burned to the ground, leaving behind a graveyard of black wooden stakes floating in a sea of grey. But the trees will grow back; new plants too. Already, fresh green shoots are sprouting up out of the ashes.

There's peace again in the Real World, though it's a much different island than it was two weeks ago. And with a bunch of London Toppers and Conqips making Box Hill their new home now, too, life is definitely going to change around here. But like we always say: different is good. Sometimes, change can be okay, too.

Before, we used to think life was perfect. But was it? If Moojag hadn't come found us, and we didn't discover Gajoomdom, we wouldn't have gotten Gran or Mum back! Gran says bad things always pass, and anyway, without the bad stuff we wouldn't appreciate the good nearly as much. She says we're all connected, and that 'opposites attract'. Well, I can't imagine our lives without Uncle Aldon in it. Who would've imagined we'd become friends? That we were even related! And Adam and Izzy got their families back, too.

And Mum's right about good things happening to you when you do good. When I went back down to Gajoomdoom for Moojag, even though I was scared, it brought her back to us, too, and in the end Moojag came home as well.

The Conqips did a lot of awful things, but they turned it around. Brix owned up to what he did wrong and even went off to live with his mum and dad! He didn't know we were watching, but he cried when he finally let Stella give him a hug. He even teamed up with the Conqips and Pofs to fill up all the boreholes and tunnels. They worked for days, filling them with cement and soil, before planting all the tree saplings from Shenbie's secret orange tree farm. So now I know that, even when you make a mistake, you can make things right again.

Who'd have thought Travis and Aldon would live with us neurodivergents, and even take up PIE crafting! Carefully guided by the Auts, of course. Once a week, they even deliver 'sweet fruits' to the Pofs. Sometimes Orange Pof and Kitty make Travis and Aldon dance for them, which seems a bit rude. But they don't seem to mind, and I guess a little friendly payback can't hurt. Aldon still groans about PIE, even though it helps him walk when his knees give in, and keeps his meltdowns away. Travis really loves his, though. I don't think he'll ever tire of asking Spondylux about the history of his name. Spondylux probably will, though!

And just when I thought I'd got my long-lost brother back, he decides to move to the forest 'for life'. Everyone accepted his choice, of course, to be alone and live like a sloth. Dad says it's our 'unconditional love' that lets him go. Does that mean, whatever Moojag does, and however far away he is, we'll always love him? And even though he's brave and strong, he knows we'll always be there for him, if he ever needs our help?

Mum says 'absence makes the heart grow fonder'—but I don't think my bursting *kardia* has a molecule of space left in it. Hopefully, at some point, he'll get bored of his own company.

I rest my head on Moojag's shoulder, and peer round at Marcel. That's definitely a happy grin. I smile and look back at the sky, changing with every moment, as we see in the new day. Not just any new day—a new day in a new, ever better, Real World, where everyone can finally live together, or apart, as one.

Moojag nods and, without a sound, speaks our words—*Imagine...*

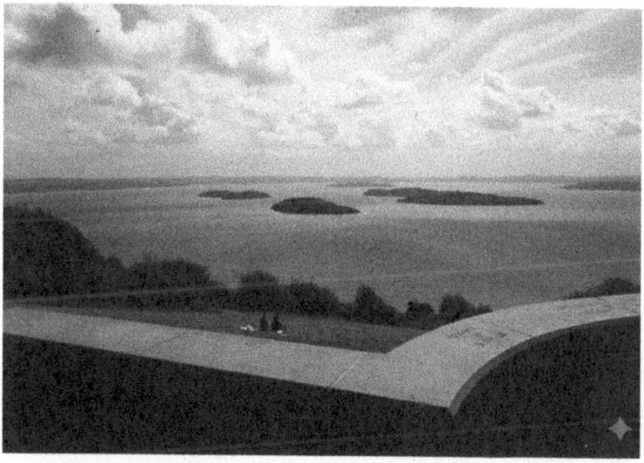

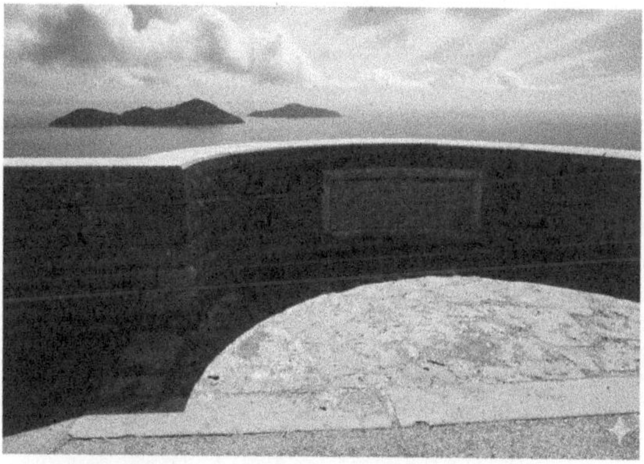

Photo: *Box Hill Viewpoint at Salomons Memorial*

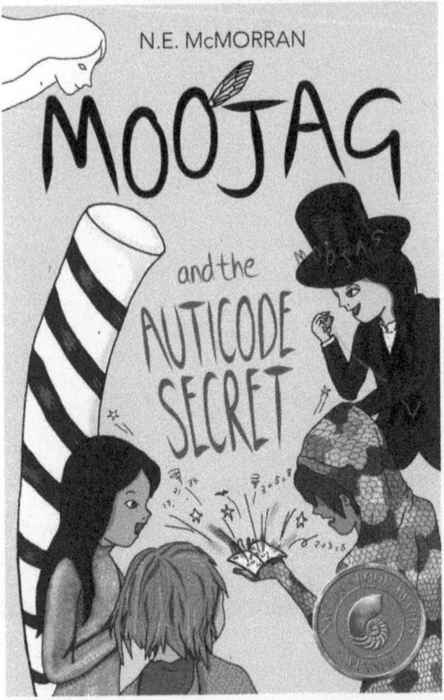
N.E. McMORRAN
MOOJAG
and the
AUTICODE
SECRET

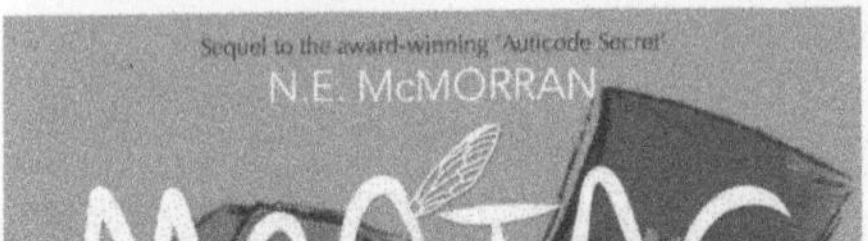
Sequel to the award-winning 'Auticode Secret'
N.E. McMORRAN
MOOJAG
and the
LOST MEMORIES
'Fantastical fun... Go grannies!' Patience Agbabi The Leap Cycle